Workbook for
Step-by-Step
Medical Coding

2 0 0 7   E D I T I O N

Carol J. Buck, MS, CPC, CPC-H, CCS-P

Program Director, Retired
Medical Secretary Programs
Northwest Technical College
East Grand Forks, Minnesota

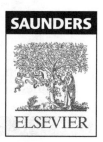

SAUNDERS

ELSEVIER

ELSEVIER
SAUNDERS

11830 Westline Industrial Drive
St. Louis, Missouri 63146

WORKBOOK FOR STEP-BY-STEP MEDICAL CODING   ISBN-13: 978-1-4160-0137-9
                                                   ISBN-10: 1-4160-0137-9

Notice

Knowledge and best practice in this field are constantly changing. As new research and
experience broaden our knowledge, changes in practice, treatment and drug therapy may
become necessary or appropriate. Readers are advised to check the most current information
provided (i) on procedures featured or (ii) by the manufacturer of each product to be
administered, to verify the recommended dose or formula, the method and duration of
administration, and contraindications. It is the responsibility of the practitioner, relying on
their own experience and knowledge of the patient, to make diagnoses, to determine
dosages and the best treatment for each individual patient, and to take all appropriate safety
precautions. To the fullest extent of the law, neither the Publisher nor the Author assumes
any liability for any injury and/or damage to persons or property arising out of or related to
any use of the material contained in this book.

The Publisher

ISBN-13: 978-1-4160-0137-9
ISBN-10: 1-4160-0137-9

Acquisitions Editor: Michael Ledbetter
Associate Developmental Editor: Josh Rapplean
Publishing Services Manager: Melissa Lastarria
Designer: Andrea Lutes

Printed in the United States of America

Last digit is the print number: 9 8 7 6 5 4 3 2 1

Collaborators and Reviewers

TECHNICAL COLLABORATOR

Jody Klitz, CPC
Business Transaction Specialist
Cancer Center of North Dakota
Grand Forks, North Dakota

REVIEWER

Jacqueline Klitz Grass, MA, CPC
Business Manager/Reimbursement Coding
The Kidney and Hypertension Center
Grand Forks, North Dakota

Preface

LET THIS BE YOUR GOAL:

People who have accomplished worthwhile [goals] have had a very high sense of the way to do things. They have not been content with mediocrity. They have not confined themselves to the beaten tracks; they have never been satisfied to do things just as others do them, but always a little better. They always pushed things that came to their hands a little higher up, a little farther on. It is this little higher up, this little farther on, that counts in the quality of life's work. It is the constant effort to be first class in everything one attempts that conquers the heights of excellence.

Orison Swett Marden

This *Workbook* has been developed to assist you in the application of the theoretical and practical coding knowledge presented in the textbook *Step-by-Step Medical Coding*. The *Workbook* parallels the textbook with presentation of Chapters 1 through 16 and includes ample opportunity to practice the skill of medical coding. The *Workbook* contains three levels of questions—theory, abbreviated patient service and diagnosis descriptions, and original reports. The first level of question is the theory question; these questions are fill-in-the-blanks, multiple choice, true or false, and matching and often include medical terminology based on the specific area of coding presented in the coding manuals. The theory information serves as the foundational knowledge necessary to correctly code services and diagnoses. The second level of question is the abbreviated patient service and diagnosis descriptions; these questions begin the practical application of coding. The descriptions are condensed statements that provide broad-based coding experience. The final level is presented at the end of each *Workbook* chapter along with reports that represent more complex services and diagnosis descriptions, such as operative, pathology, radiology, and emergency services.

The format for student answers has been developed to guide students in the development of their coding ability by using a format that includes four response variations:

- One answer blank for coding questions that require one code for the answer
- Multiple answer blanks for coding questions that require more than one code for the answer
- Key terms next to the blank(s) to guide students through the most difficult coding scenarios
- Answer blanks with 🌐 preceding the blank to indicate that the student must decide the number of codes necessary to correctly answer the question

Appendix B of the *Workbook* contains the answers to the odd-numbered questions. It is very important that you first complete the questions and then check your answers. The skill of medical coding can be acquired only through practice and by learning from mistakes that we all make along the way. It is from the understanding of why a service or diagnosis is coded in a certain way that you will develop a strong foundation that will serve you well throughout your coding career. Always take the time to read each code description fully, all notes connected with the code, and any applicable guidelines.

It is my sincere hope that you find the material presented in the *Workbook* challenging, enlightening, and worth your time and effort. Do your very best and it will show in the quality of your work.

Carol J. Buck, MS, CPC, CPC-H, CCS-P

Contents

CHAPTER 1

Introduction to the CPT

THEORY

Without the use of reference material, complete the following:

There were six index location methods presented in Chapter 1. List any four of the methods.

1. _Service or Procedure_
2. _anatomic site_
3. _Condition or disease_
4. _Synonym, eponym, abbreviation_

Match the appendix with the information it contains.

5. __D__ Appendix H   a. Modifier -63 Information on Infants <4 kg

6. __a__ Appendix F   b. Moderate Sedation

7. __b__ Appendix G   c. Genetic Testing Modifiers

8. __c__ Appendix I   d. Descriptions of Category II codes

9. You would expect to find the CPT code 71010 in what section of the CPT manual?

Radiology

10. What is the report called that a physician dictates to show that an unusual or rare procedure is performed?

    Special report

11. What association publishes the CPT?

    AMA American Medical Ass.

12. When you see the symbol ▲ in front of a code, you know what about the code?

    changed, revised, modified

13. What type of code has the full code description?

    stand-alone code

14. What type of code has only a portion of the code description?

    indented

15. What would providers enter on the insurance form to show payers which services were performed?

    CPT Codes

16. The use of a coding system allows you to communicate not only quickly, but also: _efficiently_

17. The first edition of the CPT was published in what year? _1966_

18. The updated CPT manual is published in what month? _November_

19. A standard for communicating health care data, as represented in CPT-5, was necessary to address requirements of this 1996 act:

    HIPPA Health Insurance

    Portability and _Accountability_ Act.

20. What does the symbol of a circle with a line through it (⊘) placed before a CPT code indicate about the code?

    -51 exempt code

○ **PRACTICAL**

With the use of the CPT manual section guidelines, identify the following unlisted codes:

Radiology

21. Clinical brachytherapy — 77799

22. Therapeutic radiology clinical treatment planning 77299 *Radiation Therapy, Planning*

23. Therapeutic radiology treatment management 77499

Pathology and Laboratory

24. Surgical pathology procedure 88399 (Pathology Surgical unlisted Services + Procedures

25. Urinalysis procedure 81099

Medicine

26. Allergy/clinical immunological service 95199

27. Special dermatological service 96999

28. Dialysis procedures, inpatient or outpatient 90999 (Dialysis, Unlisted Services + Procedures)

PRACTICAL

With the use of the CPT manual section guidelines, identify the following unlisted codes:

Radiology

21. Clinical brachytherapy _— 77799_

22. Therapeutic radiology clinical treatment planning _77299_ *Radiation Therapy, Planning*

23. Therapeutic radiology treatment management _77499_

Pathology and Laboratory

24. Surgical pathology procedure _88399 (Pathology, Surgical, unlisted Services + Procedures_

25. Urinalysis procedure _81099_

Medicine

26. Allergy/clinical immunological service _95199_

27. Special dermatological service _96999_

28. Dialysis procedures, inpatient or outpatient _90999_ *(Dialysis, Unlisted Services + Procedures)*

CHAPTER 2

Evaluation and Management (E/M) Section

THEORY

Without the use of reference material, complete the following:

1. _____ Consultation

2. _____ Admission

3. _____ Office visit

4. _____ Newborn care

5. _____ Established patient

6. _____ Inpatient

7. _____ New patient

8. _____ Outpatient

a. A face-to-face encounter in an office between the physician and patient

b. One who has not received services from the physician or another physician in the same group within the last 3 years

c. Advice or opinion from one physician to another physician

d. One who has been formally admitted to an acute health care facility

e. One who has received services from the physician or another physician in the same group within the last 3 years

f. Attention to an acute illness or injury that results in hospitalization

g. Evaluation and determination of care for a newborn infant

h. One who has not been formally admitted to a health care facility

The four types of medical decision making, in order of complexity from most to least complex, are as follows:

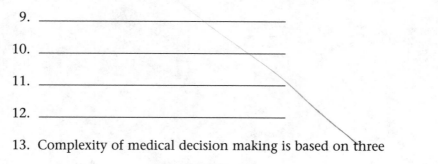

9. _____

10. _____

11. _____

12. _____

13. Complexity of medical decision making is based on three

   _____

List the five types of presenting problems from the most risk and least recovery to least risk and most recovery:

14. _____

15. _____

16. _____

17. _____

18. _____

19. Counseling and coordination of care are what kind of factors in most cases?

   _____

20. Time that is used as a guide for outpatient services is what kind of time?

   _____

   Inpatient time spent at the bedside or nursing station during or after the visit is what kind of time? _____

21. The patient's _____ _____ will reflect the number of systems examined by a brief statement of the findings.

22. A discussion with a patient and/or family concerning one or more of the following areas: diagnostic results, impressions, and/or recommended diagnostic studies; prognosis; risks and benefits of treatment; instructions for treatment; importance of compliance with treatment; risk factor reduction; and patient and family education is

   _____.

23. The history is the _____ information the patient tells the physician.

24. There is no distinction made between the new and established patients in this service department of a hospital:

_____

25. Those services rendered by a physician whose opinion or advice is requested by another physician or agency in the evaluation and/or

treatment of a patient is a _____, whereas the physician who has primary responsibility for the patient in the hospital is called

_____.

26. When critically ill patients in medical emergencies require the constant attendance of the physician (e.g., cardiac arrest, shock, bleeding, and respiratory failure) to stabilize them, what kind of care is needed?

_____

27. When care is provided for similar services (e.g., hospital visits) to the same patient by more than one physician on the same day for different conditions, the care is

_____.

28. What is the name for the transfer of the total or specific care of a patient from one physician to another that does not constitute a consultation?

_____

29. An inventory of body systems obtained through questioning to identify signs and/or symptoms that the patient may be experiencing is a

_____ of _____.

30. If the physician who is standing by does so for 25 minutes, can he or she round the time up to 30 minutes for reporting purposes?

_____

PRACTICAL

Office or Other Outpatient Services and Hospital Inpatient Service

With the use of the CPT manual, complete the following:

31. Analyze this case in which the patient record states: 40-year-old male patient (new) is evaluated for contusion of a finger. The history and examination were problem focused.

    a. Diagnosis and management options for contusion of finger. (Options can be minimal, limited, multiple, or extensive). Diagnosis and

    management options: _____

    Data to review to provide service. (Data can be minimal/none, limited, moderate, or extensive.) Only data available are current information

    obtained during the visit. Data: _____

    b. Risks if left untreated. (Risk can be minimal, low, moderate, or high.)

    Risks: _____

    c. All three of the elements have been met to qualify this patient for what level of decision-making complexity?

    _____

    d. The patient record indicates that a problem-focused history and examination were done. When this is combined with the level of decision-making complexity you arrived at for this patient, what is the correct CPT code for the case? Code(s):

    _____

32. A patient who was on observation status for 48 hours is discharged from the hospital. Code only the discharge services.

    Code: 99217 (E/M, Hospital Services, Observation Care)

33. Initial observation of a patient was for upper abdominal pain, dizziness, and anemia. A comprehensive history and examination was performed. Moderate complexity decision making was conducted to admit the patient to observation to treat and rule out causes of the patient's anemia.

    Code: 99219 (Evaluation & Management, Hospital Services Observation)

34. A 16-year-old female is being admitted by her family practice physician with a 2-week history of fatigue and fever. It has been progressively getting worse. She is also suffering from dehydration. The physician performs a comprehensive history to look for explanations for her fatigue, including recent activity level and recent sleep habits. A detailed examination is performed and she is diagnosed with mononucleosis and admitted for treatment.

    Code: 99221 (Hospital Services, Inpatient Services, Initial Hospital Care)

35. A 56-year-old male with an established history of ASHD and past stent placement is admitted through the emergency room with acute chest pain. An EKG was performed and troponin levels taken. Both showed evidence of the patient having an acute inferior wall myocardial infarction. The cardiologist performs a comprehensive history, with the chief complaint, 4 from the history of present illness (HPI), a complete review of systems (ROS), and past, family, and, social history (PFSH). The history includes the information that the pain started a week ago but last night worsened. Also on a scale of 1 to 10, he rated the pain an 8. It was also discovered that the patient has not been attending regular appointments in the clinic setting. A comprehensive examination was performed along with high-complexity medical decision making (MDM), including management of the patient's acute MI and reviewing data of the medical history of the patient. He was taken immediately to the cardiac catheterization lab to look for the source for the patient's MI.

    Code: _99223 (Hospital Services, Inpatient Services, Initial Hosp. Care_

36. The patient is a 34-year-old established patient seen in the clinic by her dermatologist. She is followed for extensive psoriasis involving her scalp, trunk, and arms. It has now worsened and spread to her palms, and she is now also complaining of joint pain. The spread to her hands has made it difficult to do many of her day-to-day tasks. A detailed history and examination are performed. The examination includes inspection of the affected areas in addition to bending and rotation of joints. A long discussion took place regarding a change in her medications to try to gain better control of her psoriasis and slow down the systemic progression. Topical and systemic treatment was decided on.

    Code(s): _99214 (E/M, Office & Other Outpatient_

37. A 2-year-old boy with bacterial pneumonia is hospitalized and has had 5 days of antibiotic therapy. Today the child developed a fever of 101° F with a mild rash on his torso. In a subsequent hospital visit, the attending physician performed a problem-focused history and examination. The MDM complexity was low.

    Code(s): _99231 (Hospital Service, Inpatient Service, Subsequent Hospital Care_

38. The patient is a 52-year-old male from out of state visiting his daughter. He left his medications for his hypertension at home and is now here in the clinic in need of a prescription. A problem-focused history and examination is performed and a prescription is given to the patient.

    Code(s): _99201 (E/M, Office & Other Outpatient)_

Consultation Services

39. A 47-year-old female was sent by her family practice physician for an office consultation with a gynecologist. The patient has been suffering with moderate pelvic pain, a heavy sensation in her lower pelvis, and marked discomfort during sexual intercourse. In a detailed history, the gynecologist noted the location, severity, and duration of her pelvic pain and related symptoms. In the review of systems, the patient had

positive findings related to her gastrointestinal, genitourinary, and endocrine body systems. The physician noted that her medical history was noncontributory to the present problem. The detailed physical examination centered on her gastrointestinal and genitourinary systems, with a complete pelvic examination. The physician ordered laboratory tests and a pelvic ultrasound to determine uterine fibroids, endometritis, or other internal gynecological pathology. The MDM complexity was moderate.

Code: 99243

40. This is a 38-year-old female with severe low back pain due to an injury she experienced as a factory worker 4 years ago. The pain has become almost unbearable, and her internal medicine physician cannot go any further with her treatment. An initial outpatient consultation is requested and the patient is sent to see the pain management specialist for suggestions to control the pain. A comprehensive history is taken, including all of the pertinent information regarding her injury. During the comprehensive examination the patient's gait and movement were observed. Moderate-complexity decision making is performed, including different treatment options. A separate note is dictated to show the requesting physician what results were found during the visit and the decision on treatment of her pain.

Code: 99244 (Consultation, office +/or other Outpatient

41. An inpatient urological consultation is performed for a 32-year-old female who recently had an elective abortion performed on an outpatient basis. The woman has been admitted with a high fever, pelvic pain, and dysuria. During a detailed history, the urologist notes in the history of present illness that the patient's symptoms began about 2 days after the abortion and progressed to the acute phase, which she is in at the present time. The location of the pain is in the lower abdomen and rated 9 on a scale of 1 to 10. She reports the quality of the pain to be sharp and stabbing. In the review of systems, the physician notes positive responses in 5 of the 12 body systems investigated. The urologist notes a negative medical history related to urinary symptoms other than a mild cystitis about 10 years ago. The detailed physical examination performed by the urologist centers on the genitourinary system and gastrointestinal system in significant detail. The medical decision making is low. Given the patient's past surgical procedure and physical findings at the present, the consultant considers the diagnoses of pyelonephritis, cystitis, pyelitis, and endometritis.

Code: 99253 (NP, Initial Inpatient Consultation

42. A 46-year-old male is admitted to the hospital with a progressive staphylococcal pneumonia that is not responding to treatment. A request is made for the infectious disease physician on staff to render his opinion for treatment. The patient is seen in initial inpatient consultation. An expanded problem-focused history and examination are performed. After looking at the sputum cultures, the physician decides on the most effective antibiotic for treatment. The decision making is straightforward.

Code: 99252 (NP, Initial Inpatient Consultation)

43. The initial consulting physician subsequently sees a 55-year-old patient injured at work when he fell from a house roof and struck his head. The patient had a right frontal parietal craniotomy 6 days previously and is recovering rapidly. The initial consultation was requested regarding a drug reaction that produced a rash on the upper torso. The consultant recommended a medication change, but after 48 hours the patient had no improvement. The physician reevaluates for other possible causes of the rash. An expanded problem-focused interval history and a physical examination were performed. The MDM complexity was moderate.

    Code: _99232 (Hosp. Inpatient Service, Subsequent Hosp. Care_

44. A 44-year-old patient, with chronic mastoiditis, was seen in consultation by the ENT specialist in the office. Her physician was inquiring as to the advantages of surgery versus continued antibiotic treatment when an acute flare comes on. The ENT specialist recommends surgery because of the increasing severity with each acute flare. She is fearful of the surgery because of the need to go under general anesthetic and a fear of permanent hearing loss. The physician performs an expanded problem-focused history to include the duration of this problem and how many acute flares a year the patient experiences. An expanded problem-focused examination and straightforward decision making is completed. It is determined that with the number of acute flares a year and the increasing severity of each case that surgery is recommended. The patient's fears are laid to rest and the patient decides to go ahead with the surgery.

    Code: _99242 (Office Consultation, New or Established Patient)_

45. This is a follow-up visit on a 28-year-old male who is admitted with the diagnosis of headaches. The patient is subsequently seen because the physician needs to follow-up on test results that weren't back yet at the initial consultation. This will help to find a possible cause of the headaches and course of treatment. A problem-focused history and examination and low-complexity decision making is made after viewing the CT results. The diagnosis of tension headaches was made and treatment options discussed.

    Code(s): _99231 (Hospital Inpatient Service, Subsequent Hosp. Care)_

46. An 83-year-old patient is seen at the local nursing home. The patient suffers from severe COPD. Routine labs were drawn on the patient by her primary doctor and her blood sugar came back abnormal. Fasting glucose was then taken and was high. The endocrinologist was asked to render an opinion on a possible diagnosis of diabetes. A problem-focused history and examination, and straightforward decision making was made. Diabetes was diagnosed and treatment started. The endocrinologist contacted the primary physician and discussed treatment of the patient.

    Code(s): _99251 (Consultation, Inpatient, New Established Patient_

47. A patient is sent to a general surgeon by her family physician for an opinion and recommendation for surgical repair of a hernia. A brief

problem-focused history of present illness and a problem-focused examination of the affected body area and organ system are performed in the office. The MDM complexity was straightforward.

Code(s): _99241 (Office Consult. New Establish Patient_

48. A pulmonologist is asked, by the patient's primary physician, to see a 14-month-old boy, who was admitted to the hospital with respiratory distress, cough, and fever. A comprehensive history is taken from the parents because this is an infant. It was determined that the patient does attend a day care facility. The cough and fever have been going on for approximately 5 days. The infant started having trouble breathing just this morning. The patient is intubated. Pneumonia is the standing diagnosis. A comprehensive examination is performed along with moderate decision making. More tests will follow. A copy of his dictation will be sent to the primary physician.

Code(s): _99254 (New Patient, Initial inpatient Consult._

49. Office consultation is requested by workers' compensation for a 32-year-old man on workers' compensation who is unable to work because of a dislocated vertebra. Two previous surgical repairs have been unsuccessful in relieving the patient's pain. The patient has been unable to return to his employment as a bricklayer. He complains of radiating pain throughout the buttocks and leg, with numbness throughout the leg and foot. Reflexes are minimal to nonexistent. A second opinion is being asked from a neurosurgeon to confirm or refute previous treatment plans. A comprehensive history and physical examination are performed. MDM complexity was high due to the prior surgeries and continued complaints.

Code(s): _99245 (Office Consultation, New/Establish Patient_

Emergency Department Services, Nursing Facility, Domiciliary, and Home Services

50. A patient presents to the emergency department after being involved in a motor vehicle accident. The patient was wearing a seat belt. The vehicle rolled numerous times. The patient's head struck the side window. The patient is unresponsive and is intubated. A history was unable to be obtained because of the patient's unresponsiveness. What history is available comes from the paramedics and patient's record. A comprehensive examination reveals the abdomen to be quite swollen with extensive bruising around the lower abdomen caused by the seat belt. High-complexity decision making was involved and the patient was rushed to the operating room.

Code: _99285 (EMS Services)_

51. A male patient presents to the emergency department with a wrist sprain sustained in a softball game when the patient slid into home. The patient is in apparent pain with a swollen wrist, which he is unable to flex. An expanded problem-focused history and physical examination are done. Radiographs show a fracture of the distal radius. The MDM complexity was low.

Code: _99281 (Emergency Department services_

52. The 88-year-old female's family physician comes to the nursing facility to perform the resident's annual assessment. A detailed interval history is taken with some information from the patient, but because of her limited cognitive abilities, most of the information is gathered from the nurses and past records. A comprehensive multisystem physical examination is performed, which includes extensive body areas and related organ systems. The MDM complexity was low because multiple diagnoses must be considered for this patient, who has senile dementia, diabetes, hypertension, hypothyroidism, and recurrent transient ischemic attacks. The creation of a new treatment plan is required because some of the patient's conditions have worsened.

   Code: _____

53. This is a home visit on an elderly gentleman who is complaining of swelling in his lower extremities. Pain is associated with this. An expanded problem-focused history and examination are performed and low-complexity decision making. Jobst stockings are prescribed.

   Code: _99318_ *All three components must be met - Typically would be appended to this level because consent was required by Worker's comp -32 Modifier*

54. Subsequent follow-up care is provided for the 82-year-old male nursing facility patient with Alzheimer's disease. The resident has responded well to some new medications and appears to have recovered some of his cognitive abilities. The physician performs a problem-focused history and physical examination on his neurological problem and orders the current treatments continued. The MDM complexity is low.

   Code(s): _____

55. Subsequent follow-up care is provided for the patient who was transferred to a nursing facility from an acute care hospital after partial recovery from a stroke. The patient has developed periods of extreme dizziness and mental confusion. A detailed interval history is gathered, and a detailed physical examination of the affected body systems is performed. Given the possibility that a new stroke could have occurred or that other neurological problems have developed, new orders are written, and the physician plans to return the next day to evaluate the patient's condition again. The MDM complexity is moderate.

   Code(s): _____

56. The physician provides services to a resident of a rest home for an ulcerative sore on the foot. Given the fact that the patient is in reasonably good health and is not diabetic, the physician focuses his attention on the right lower extremity during the problem-focused physical examination. The physician knows the resident well and performs a brief HPI and ROS during a problem-focused history. The resident thinks the sore is from new shoes recently purchased, and the physician agrees with that conclusion. Topical antibiotic cream is ordered, and the new shoes are sent to the cobbler to be stretched. The MDM complexity is straightforward.

   Code(s): _____

57. The physician provides services to a new patient who is in a custodial care center. The patient is a 43-year-old paraplegic who has severe infected stasis ulcers. The physician performs a detailed history and examination, and prescribes an antibiotic. The MDM was straightforward.

   Code(s): _____

Prolonged Services and Preventative Medicine

58. An established patient is seen in the office for a new problem that requires a comprehensive history and examination. The MDM complexity is high, and the physician spends 40 minutes with the patient. However, the patient has numerous concerns, and the physician spends an additional hour and 50 minutes in prolonged direct patient contact.

   Code(s): _____   _____

   _____

59. A 44-year-old asthmatic patient (new) is scheduled for a routine office visit for a complaint of severe headaches. The physician provides a comprehensive history and examination. The MDM complexity was high. Toward the end of the visit, the patient develops severe breathing complications, and the physician spends the next hour and 30 minutes administering treatment.

   Code(s): _____

60. A 64-year-old man arrives at his appointment with his family physician for his annual physical examination. The patient has no new complaints and all of his medications remain the same. He is told to follow-up in 1 year or sooner if necessary.

   Code(s): _____

Services from Throughout the E/M Section

61. A new patient is seen in the office for a variety of medical problems. The patient has insulin-dependent diabetes mellitus with complicating eye and renal problems. She also has hypertensive heart disease with episodes of congestive heart failure. Her peripheral vascular disease has worsened, and she can walk only a block before she is crippled with extreme leg pain. The patient reports that a new problem has surfaced: throbbing headaches with radiating neck pain. To manage and investigate the multiplicity of problems, the physician performs a comprehensive history and physical examination. A complete review of systems is performed, as is an update to her complete past, family, and social history. The physician has to take a multitude of factors into consideration because this patient's problems are highly complex.

   Code: _____

62. A new patient is seen in the office complaining of a sore throat and reports a low-grade fever for the past 4 days. The physician performs an expanded problem-focused history and an expanded problem-focused

examination of the respiratory and lymphatic system. The physician's impression was pharyngitis and straightforward decision making was performed. Amoxicillin was prescribed.

Code: _____

63. This is a 32-year-old female patient admitted for observation after an allergic reaction to her pain medication. She is alert and oriented, but has severe pruritus and shortness of breath. A detailed history and examination is performed after she takes medication for the pruritus; the breathing improved and the patient was discharged from observation on the same day.

Code: _____

64. The patient was admitted to the hospital 3 days ago with severe dehydration and hypothermia. The patient is now being discharged. Discharge takes 30 minutes.

Code: _____

65. A family practice physician who is treating a 20-year-old man (inpatient) for bronchitis calls in a urologist to examine the patient, who has requested a circumcision. The consultant performs a problem-focused history and problem-focused physical examination and determines that there is no urgency for the surgical procedure. The physician's decision making is fairly straightforward, and he recommends that the patient have the procedure done as an outpatient at a later date.

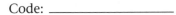 Code(s): _____

66. A physician visits a 75-year-old female in the extended nursing facility as part of her annual assessment. The physician completes a detailed interval history with a comprehensive, head-to-toe physical examination. The physician reviews and affirms the medical plan of care developed by the multidisciplinary care team at the nursing facility. The patient's condition is stable; her hypertension and diabetes (type 2) are in good control and she has no new problems. The physician has limited data to review and few diagnoses to consider. The MDM complexity was low.

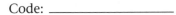 Code(s): _____

67. A 67-year-old female is admitted with severe exacerbation of her COPD. The patient is now in respiratory failure and CHF. The patient is intubated and unconscious; 155 minutes of critical care time was spent at bedside and coordinating care for this patient.

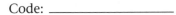 Code(s): _____

68. Henry Green, an established patient, came into the office for his yearly physical examination. Henry is 72 and in good health.

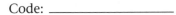 Code(s): _____

REPORTS

Toward the end of this textbook, you will find a section titled Reports, which contains original reports. Read the reports indicated below and supply the appropriate CPT code on the following lines:

69. Report 1 Code: _____

70. Report 2 Code: _____

71. Report 3 Code: _____

72. Report 4 🌑 Code(s): _____

73. Report 5 🌑 Code(s): _____

CHAPTER 3

Anesthesia Section and Modifiers

THEORY

Without the use of reference material, answer the following:

1. What two words describe a decreased level of consciousness that does not put patients completely to sleep and that allows the patients to breathe on their own during a surgical procedure?

   _____

   _____

2. What do the initials CRNA stand for?

   _____

3. What appendix in the CPT manual contains a complete list of all modifiers?

   _____

4. What is the word that means assigning multiple codes when one code would do?

   _____

5. What is the term that describes the services provided to a patient by the physician before surgery?

   _____

6. What is another term for the time after the surgery that the physician provides services to the patient?

_____

7. Do all third-party payers recognize all modifiers as listed in the CPT manual?

_____

8. What is the term that describes two physicians working together in the completion of a procedure when each has the same level of responsibility?

_____

PRACTICAL

With the use of the CPT manual, identify the following physical status modifiers.

9. Patient with a severe systemic disease that is a constant threat to life.

   Code(s): ___P4___

10. Normal healthy patient.

    Code(s): ___P1___

11. Patient with a severe systemic disease.

    Code(s): ___P3___

12. Declared brain-dead patient whose organs are being removed for donor purposes.

    Code(s): ___P6___

13. Patient with mild systemic disease.

    Code(s): ___P2___

14. Moribund patient who is not expected to survive without the operation.

    Code(s): ___P5___

Locate anesthesia procedures in the CPT manual index under the entry "anesthesia" and then subtermed by the anatomic site. Write the CPT index location on the line provided (e.g., anesthesia, thyroid). Then locate the code(s) identified in the anesthesia section of the CPT manual. Choose the correct code(s) and write the code(s) on the line provided.

15. Diagnostic arthroscopic procedure of knee joint

    Index location: ___Anesthia, Knee___

    Code: ___01382___

16. Radical hysterectomy

    Index location: ___Anesthesia, Hysterectomy, Radical___

    Code: ___00846___

17. Corneal transplant

    Index location: ___Anesthia, Corneal Transplant___

    Code: ___00144___

___18. Cesarean delivery only

Index location: _Anesthesia Cesarean Deli._

Code: _01961_

19. Otoscopy used in procedure for middle ear

Index location: _Anesthesia Otoscopy_

Code: _00124_

___20. Transurethral resection of the prostate

Index location: _Anesthesia, Transurethral Procedure_

Code: _00914_

Using the CPT manual, indicate the modifiers that would be used for the following:

21. A patient is admitted and has bilateral arthroscopy of the knees.

Modifier: _-50_

___22. Ben Carter, surgical resident, assists Dr. Wells, chief cardiologist, in a coronary artery bypass procedure. What modifier would be submitted to report Ben's services?

Modifier(s): _None - Residents Not paid_

23. Dr. Wells began surgery on an 86-year-old female with severe hypertension. The patient was satisfactorily anesthetized and the site opened to view. Shortly thereafter, the patient's blood pressure dropped significantly, and the physician was unable to stabilize the patient. The procedure was discontinued.

Modifier: _-53_

___24. The patient is a 10-month-old boy who fell while trying to walk. He cut the bottom of his lip open. Sutures are necessary but due to the patient's age and excessive movement general anesthesia is needed.

Modifier: _-23_

25. A radiological examination of the gastrointestinal tract was ordered by a third-party payer.

Modifier: _-32_

26. Anesthesia provided by the ENT physician during a tympanoplasty.

Modifier: _-47_

27. A patient is seen at the direction of Workers' Compensation for a complete physical examination.

    Modifier: _____

28. The patient returns to the operating room for removal of deep pins during the postoperative period after an open repair of a humerus fracture.

    Modifier: _____

29. A patient has a surgical procedure on Tuesday, and later that day the physician must take the patient back to the operating room for a related procedure.

    Modifier: _____

30. The patient underwent a bilateral tympanoplasty.

    Modifier: _____

31. If you must use two or more modifiers to describe a service, you would use which modifier to indicate this circumstance?

    Modifier: _____

32. A surgeon performs a procedure on a neonate weighing 9 kg; the procedure was extremely complicated. What modifier would you use to indicate this service, which has an increased level of complexity?

    Modifier: _____

33. Dr. Storely, a general surgeon, performs the preoperative and intraoperative services for a patient and the patient leaves town on a personal emergency. The patient's daughter's physician handles the postoperative management of the patient. What modifier would you use to indicate the patient's daughter's physician's services?

    Modifier: _____

34. Dr. Merideth serves as an assistant surgeon to Dr. Taylor. What modifier would you add to the procedure code to indicate Dr. Merideth's status during the procedure?

    Modifier: _____

35. The third-party payer requires the use of HCPCS/National modifiers; the surgeon performed a surgical procedure on the patient's left thumb. What Level II modifier would indicate the left thumb?

    Modifier: _____

36. What Level II modifier indicates the upper left eyelid?

    Modifier: _____

REPORTS

Toward the end of this textbook, you will find a section titled Reports, which contains original reports. Read the reports indicated below and supply the appropriate CPT anesthesia code on the following lines:

37. Report 10 Code: _____

38. Report 14 Code: _____

39. Report 15 Code: _____

40. Report 16 Code: _____

41. Report 28 Code: _____

CHAPTER 4

Surgery Section and Integumentary System

THEORY

General Medical Terminology

Without the use of reference material, match the following terms to the correct definitions.

1. __D__ Abscess

2. __F__ Benign

3. __E__ Cyst

4. __A__ Lesion

5. __B__ Malignant

6. __C__ Tumor

a. Abnormal or altered tissue (e.g., wound or boil)

b. Term used to describe a cancerous tumor that grows worse over time

c. Swelling or enlargement; a spontaneous growth of tissue that forms an abnormal mass

d. Localized collection of pus that will result in the disintegration of tissue over time

e. Closed sac containing matter or fluid

f. Not progressive or recurrent; usually used to describe a growth that does not spread to another location in the body

Match the following ways to obtain a biopsy specimen with the current definitions:

7. __C__ Aspiration

8. __D__ Punch

9. __A__ Incisional

10. __B__ Excisional

a. Surgically cutting into

b. Removal of an entire lesion for biopsy

c. Use of a needle and a syringe to withdraw fluid

d. Use of a small, hollow instrument to puncture a lesion

Match the following common procedures and suffixes to the current definitions:

11. __L__ Biopsy

12. __G__ Curettage

13. __C__ Drainage

14. __F__ Endoscopy

15. __D__ Excision

16. __M__ Incision

17. __H__ Injection

18. __N__ Ligation

19. __A__ Repair

20. __E__ Suture

21. __J__ -centesis

22. __K__ -ectomy

23. __O__ -otomy

24. __B__ -plasty

25. __I__ -rrhaphy

a. To remedy, replace, or heal

b. Suffix meaning technique involving molding or surgically forming

c. Free flow or withdrawal of fluids from a wound or cavity

d. Cutting or taking away

e. To unite parts by stitching them together

f. Inspection of body organs or cavities by the use of a lighted scope that may be placed through an existing opening or through a small incision

g. Scraping of a cavity using a spoon-shaped instrument

h. Forcing of a fluid into a vessel or cavity

i. Suffix meaning suturing

j. Suffix meaning puncture of a cavity

k. Suffix meaning removal of a part of all of an organ of the body

l. Removal of a small piece of living tissue for diagnostic purposes

m. Surgically cutting into

n. Binding or tying off, as in constricting blood flow of a vessel or binding fallopian tubes for sterilization

o. Suffix meaning incision into

Integumentary System Terminology

Match the following terms to the correct definitions:

26. _D_ Dermis

27. _J_ Epidermis

28. _P_ Subcutaneous

29. _N_ Incision and drainage

30. _C_ Abscess

31. _S_ Cyst

32. _M_ Debridement

33. _O n K_ Paring

34. _E_ Biopsy

35. _K n O_ Shaving

36. _A_ Excision

37. _G_ Benign

38. _R_ Malignant

39. _L_ Repair

40. _F_ Skin graft

41. _Q_ Tissue transfer

42. _H_ Destruction

43. _B_ Mast

44. _I_ Cryosurgery

a. Full-thickness removal of a lesion that may include simple closure

b. Prefix meaning breast

c. Localized collection of pus that will result in the disintegration of tissue over time

d. Second layer of skin holding blood vessels, nerve endings, sweat glands, and hair follicles

e. Removal of a small piece of living tissue for diagnostic purposes

f. Transplantation of tissue to repair a defect

g. Not progressive or recurrent

h. Killing of tissue, possibly by electrocautery, laser, chemical, or other means

i. Destruction of lesions using extreme cold

j. Outer layer of skin

k. Horizontal or transverse removal of dermal or epidermal lesions, without full-thickness excision

l. Pertains to suturing a wound

m. Cleansing of or removing dead tissue from a wound

n. To cut and withdraw fluid

o. Removal of thin layers of skin by peeling or scraping

p. Tissue below dermis, primarily fat cells that insulate the body

q. Piece of skin for grafting that is still partially attached to the original blood supply and is used to cover an adjacent wound area

r. Used to describe a cancerous tumor that grows worse over time

s. Closed sac containing matter or fluid

PRACTICAL

Using the CPT manual, code the following services:

45. Joan, an established patient, comes into the office to have an intermediate repair of a 2.6-cm wound on her right arm. A surgical tray was used.

    Code(s): 12032 _____

46. Rita, an established patient, has a 16.2 cm simple repair of the cheek. A surgical tray is used.

    Code(s): _____

47. Lisa, an established patient, has a percutaneous needle core biopsy with image guidance for a left breast mass. A surgical tray was used.

    Code(s): _____

48. What code would be used to report Mr. Jones's visit to Dr. Green 2 weeks after major surgery?

    Code: _____

49. Excision axillary hidradenitis, complex repair.

    Code: _____

50. Debridement; skin, subcutaneous, and muscle.

    Code: _____

51. Removal of tissue expander without insertion of prosthesis.

    Code: _____

52. Excision of pilonidal cyst; complicated.

    Code: _____

53. Insertion of Norplant contraceptive capsule.

    Code: _____

54. Debridement of four fingernails.

    Code(s): _____

55. Excision of 4-cm benign lesion of face (most resource intensive) and excision of 3-cm benign lesion of neck.

    Code(s): _____

56. Excision of a 2.5-cm malignant lip lesion and two malignant lesions of the chest, each 1.5 cm in diameter.

    Code(s): _____

57. Destruction by laser of three benign facial lesions.

    Code(s): _____

58. Destruction of 4.0-cm malignant lesion of the eyelid.

    Code(s): _____

59. Suzanne Osterland, a 4-year-old, is brought to the office by her father. Suzanne was playing on the swing set in the back yard when she fell approximately 5 feet from the top step of the play set. When she fell, she struck her leg on a birdbath rim and then on a pail with several garden tools protruding over the rim, sustaining 12.9-cm, 3.1-cm, and 2.1-cm lacerations of the right leg, requiring deep-layered closure accomplished after partial thickness debridement.

    Code(s): _____

60. Electrosurgical destruction of a 1.0-cm malignant lesion of the neck.

    Code(s): _____

61. Cryosurgical destruction of 10 flat warts on the hand.

    Code(s): _____

62. Laser destruction of multiple malignant lesions, as follows: 3.4 cm on right hand, 2.1 cm on left hand, 5.2 cm on right hand, 4.3 cm on left hand, 0.3 cm on right eyelid, 0.5 cm on left eyelid.

    Code(s): _____

63. Biopsy of three lesions of mucous membrane with simple closure.

    Code(s): _____

64. Bilateral blepharoplasty of upper eyelid.

    Code(s): _____

65. Initial, local treatment, first-degree burn.

    Code(s): _____

66. Mohs' micrographic surgery of arm, first stage, 4 tissue blocks.

    Code(s): _____

67. Mastotomy with drainage of deep abscess.

    Code(s): _____

REPORTS

Toward the end of this textbook, you will find a section titled Reports, which contains original reports. Read the reports indicated below and supply the appropriate CPT codes on the following lines:

68. Report 6 🐚 Code(s): _____

69. Report 7 🐚 Code(s): _____

70. Report 8 🐚 Code(s): _____

71. Report 9 🐚 Code(s): _____

72. Report 11 🐚 Code(s): _____

73. Report 12 🐚 Code(s): _____

CHAPTER 5

Musculoskeletal System

THEORY

Musculoskeletal Terminology

Without the use of reference material, match the following terms to the correct definitions:

1. _____ Closed treatment

2. _____ Open treatment

3. _____ Percutaneous

4. _____ Fracture

5. _____ Dislocation

6. _____ Manipulation

7. _____ Internal/external

8. _____ Skeletal traction

9. _____ Soft tissue

10. _____ Arthroplasty

11. _____ Arthrodesis

a. Application of force to a limb with the use of a pin, screw, wire, or clamp attached to the bone

b. Placement in a location other than the original location skeletal fixation

c. The application of pins, wires, screws, and so on to immobilize; these can be placed externally or internally

d. Fracture treatment when site is not surgically opened and visualized or reduction

e. Words used interchangeably to mean the attempted restoration of a fracture or joint fixation

f. Fracture site that is surgically opened and visualized

g. Surgical immobilization of a joint

h. Tissues (fascia, connective tissue, muscle, etc.) surrounding a bone

i. Break in a bone

j. Considered neither open nor closed; fracture is not visualized, but fixation is placed across the fracture site under x-ray imaging

k. Reshaping or reconstructing a joint

Without the use of reference material, answer the following:

12. Would a biopsy code usually include the administration of any necessary local anesthesia?

     _____

13. What is arthrocentesis? _____

     _____

14. What is a uniplane fixation device? _____

     _____

15. What is the name of the graft that is taken from the lower thigh area where the fascia is the thickest?

     _____

16. What type of stimulation often is used to promote healing of a slow-healing fracture?

     _____

17. What is fast becoming the surgical method of choice for many musculoskeletal procedures today?

     _____

18. What is the term that describes the use of tape applied to the body to provide support or limit motion?

     _____

19. Do you bill for the removal of a cast that your physician applied?

     Yes _____ No _____

20. What two words describe when elastic wrap or tape is fastened to the skin or wrapped around a limb and weights are then attached to the wraps or tape?

     _____

21. What is the primary difference between the excision codes found in the musculoskeletal system subsection and the excision codes found in the integumentary system subsection?

     _____

     _____

PRACTICAL

With the use of the CPT manual, code the following:

22. John is returning to the physician's office 2 weeks postsurgery for an application of a long leg cast.

    Code: _____

23. Julie Mason is coming in today to have her long-arm cast removed and replaced with a short-arm cast.

    Code: _____

24. Jamiee Larson slipped on the ice and twisted her knee when she fell. On diagnostic arthroscopy, a torn medial and lateral meniscus tear was seen and repaired.

    Code: _____

25. Percutaneous skeletal fixation of calcaneal fracture requiring manipulation.

    Code: _____

26. Closed treatment of a pelvic ring fracture; without manipulation.

    Code: _____

27. Closed treatment of a single metacarpophalangeal dislocation; with manipulation and without anesthesia.

    Code: _____

28. Open treatment of a traumatic hip dislocation without fixation.

    Code: _____

29. Closed treatment of a patellar fracture; no manipulation.

    Code:_____

30. Closed treatment of a patellar dislocation; no anesthesia.

    Code: _____

31. Manipulation of a knee joint under general anesthesia with application of a traction device.

    Code: _____

32. Closed treatment of a tarsal bone dislocation without anesthesia.

    Code: _____

33. Depressed frontal sinus fracture repaired using open treatment.

    Code: _____

34. Open treatment of a Lefort I maxillary fracture.

    Code: _____

35. Aspiration and injection of a bone cyst.

    Code: _____

36. Removal of deep screws from a repaired fracture.

    Code: _____

37. Replantation of index finger, including tendon insertion, following a complete traumatic amputation. Code only the replantation service.

    Code: _____

38. Costochondral cartilage graft.

    Code: _____

39. Therapeutic injection of corticosteroids for carpal tunnel.

    Code: _____

40. Aspiration of a shoulder joint.

    Code: _____

41. Removal of a halo that was applied by another physician.

    Code(s): _____

42. Subsequent removal of a short-arm cast by the physician who applied the cast.

    Code(s): _____

43. Closed treatment of a mandibular fracture without manipulation.

    Code(s): _____

44. Application of a shoulder-to-hip body cast.

    Code(s): _____

45. Wedging of a clubfoot cast.

    Code(s): _____

46. Application of a short leg splint.

    Code(s): _____

47. Strapping of a hip.

    🔊 Code(s): _____

48. Application of a long-arm splint.

    🔊 Code(s): _____

49. Strapping of a 40-year-old's low back.

    🔊 Code(s): _____

50. Surgical arthroscopy of the temporomandibular joint.

    🔊 Code(s): _____

51. Application, cast; figure-of-eight.

    🔊 Code(s): _____

52. Surgical arthroscopy, elbow; limited debridement.

    🔊 Code(s): _____

53. Diagnostic hip arthroscopy.

    🔊 Code(s): _____

54. Surgical arthroscopy with lateral meniscus repair of knee.

    🔊 Code(s): _____

55. Arthroscopic chondroplasty of knee with minimal debridement.

    🔊 Code(s): _____

56. Endoscopic plantar fasciotomy.

    🔊 Code(s): _____

57. Release of a transverse carpal ligament of the wrist with surgical endoscopy.

    🔊 Code(s): _____

58. Arthrocentesis of ganglion cyst of toe joint, both injection and aspiration.

    🔊 Code(s): _____

59. Excision of maxillary torus palatinus.

    🔊 Code(s): _____

REPORTS

Toward the end of this textbook, you will find a section titled Reports, which contains original reports. Read the reports indicated below and supply the appropriate CPT codes on the following lines:

60. Report 10 🦴 Code(s): _____

61. Report 13 🦴 Code(s): _____

62. Report 14 🦴 Code(s): _____

63. Report 15 🦴 Code(s): _____

64. Report 16 🦴 Code(s): _____

65. Report 17 🦴 Code(s): _____

66. Report 18 🦴 Code(s): _____

CHAPTER 6

Respiratory System

THEORY

Without the use of reference material, complete the following:

Respiratory Terminology

Match the following terms and prefixes to the correct definition:

1. _____ Polyp

2. _____ Rhino-

3. _____ Endoscopy

4. _____ Sinuses

5. _____ Antrum

6. _____ Antrotomy

7. _____ Laryngo-

8. _____ Bronchoscopy

9. _____ Thoracentesis

10. _____ Thoracotomy

11. _____ Thoracostomy

a. Excision of a lobe of the lung
b. Maxillary sinus
c. Prefix meaning larynx
d. Tumor on a pedicle that bleeds easily and may become malignant
e. Prefix meaning lung or air
f. Surgical puncture of the thoracic cavity, usually using a needle, to remove fluids
g. Inspection of the bronchial tree using a bronchoscope
h. Prefix meaning nose
i. Use of a lighted endoscope to view the pleural spaces and thoracic cavity or perform surgical procedures
j. Removal of blockage (embolism) from vessels
k. Inspection of body organs or cavities using a lighted scope that may be placed through an existing opening or through a small incision
l. Covering of the lungs and thoracic cavity that is moistened with serous fluid to reduce friction during respiratory movements of the lungs

12. _____ Thoracoscopy

13. _____ Lobectomy

14. _____ Pleura

15. _____ Pneumo-

16. _____ Embolectomy

m. Cutting into the thoracic cavity to allow for enlargement of the heart or for drainage

n. Cutting through the antrum wall to make an opening in the sinus

o. Cavities within the nasal bones

p. Surgical incision into the thoracic cavity

17. What is the name of the item that is placed into the hole in a deviated septum as a repair without surgical grafting? _____

_____

18. What is the name of the surgical procedure for the reshaping of the nose?

_____

19. What is the name of the surgical procedure for the rearrangement of the nasal septum often used in patients with a deviated septum?

_____

20. This term means destruction by removing, usually by cutting:

_____

21. Which approach is most difficult to control, posterior or anterior?

_____

22. What term describes washing out of an organ?

_____

23. What are the two different approaches that can be used to do tracheostomy?

_____ and _____

24. If a surgeon performs a thoracotomy procedure and at the end of the procedure inserts a chest tube for drainage, do you report the insertion of the tube separately?

_____

25. If bilateral destruction of maxillary sinuses is performed, what modifier would you use? _____

26. Removal of two lobes of a lung is termed a _____

PRACTICAL

With the use of the CPT manual, complete the following:

27. Endoscopic maxillary antrostomy with removal of granulation tissue.

    Code: _____

28. Ben is a 5-year-old who swallowed a nickel. Patient needed an indirect laryngoscopy to remove this foreign body.

    Code: _____

29. Bronchoscopy with transbronchial biopsies of two lobes of the right lung.

    Code: _____

30. Flexible bronchoscopy with brushings.

    Code: _____

31. Diagnostic flexible fiber optic laryngoscopy.

    Code: _____

32. Intranasal biopsy.

    Code: _____

33. Cauterization of superficial mucosa of bilateral inferior turbinates.

    Code: _____

34. Primary rhinoplasty with elevation of nasal tip.

    Code: _____

35. Extensive bilateral removal of nasal polyps, performed in the hospital outpatient department.

    Code(s): _____

36. Insertion of a septal button.

    Code: _____

37. Direct, operative, laryngoscopy with biopsy, with use of the operating microscope.

    Code: _____

38. Establishment and subsequent insertion of voice button.

    Code: _____

39. Arytenoidectomy; external approach.

    Code(s): _____

40. Laryngoscopy, with stroboscopy.

    Code(s): _____

41. Nasotracheal catheter aspiration.

    Code(s): _____

42. Cervical tracheoplasty.

    Code(s): _____

43. Revision of a tracheostomy scar.

    Code(s): _____

44. Pneumocentesis.

    Code(s): _____

45. Surgical thoracoscopy, with wedge resection of the lung.

    Code(s): _____

46. Double lung transplant with cardiopulmonary bypass.

    Code(s): _____

47. Repair hernia of the lung through the chest wall.

    Code(s): _____

48. Open closure of a major bronchial fistula.

    Code(s): _____

49. Therapeutic fracture of inferior nasal turbinates.

    Code(s): _____

50. Sinuostomy, sphenoid, without biopsy.

    Code(s): _____

51. Tracheostoma revision, simple, without flap rotation.

    Code(s): _____

52. Bronchial biopsy.

    Code(s): _____

53. Total pneumonectomy.

    🔗 Code(s): _____

54. Diagnostic thoracoscopy of the pericardial sac, with biopsy.

    🔗 Code(s): _____

55. Extrapleural resection of the ribs, all stages.

    🔗 Code(s): _____

56. Carinal reconstruction.

    🔗 Code(s): _____

57. Chemical pleurodesis.

    🔗 Code(s): _____

58. Excision dermoid cyst of the nose, complex.

    🔗 Code(s): _____

REPORTS

Toward the end of this textbook, you will find a section titled Reports, which contains original reports. Read the reports indicated below and supply the appropriate CPT codes on the following lines:

59. Report 19 🐚 Code(s): _____

60. Report 21 🐚 Code(s): _____

61. Report 23 🐚 Code(s): _____

62. Report 24 🐚 Code(s): _____

CHAPTER 7

—

Cardiovascular System

THEORY

Without the use of reference material, complete the following:

Cardiovascular Terminology

Match the following terms to the correct definitions:

1. _____ Pericardium

2. _____ Cardiopulmonary

3. _____ Bypass

4. _____ Pacemaker

5. _____ Single-chamber pacemaker

6. _____ Dual-chamber pacemaker

7. _____ Electrode

8. _____ Ventricle

9. _____ Atrium

10. _____ Cardioverter-defibrillator

a. Forcing of fluid into a vessel or cavity

b. Blood bypasses the heart through a heart-lung machine during open heart surgery

c. Lead attached to a generator that carries the electrical current from the generator to the atria or ventricles

d. Vessel that carries unoxygenated blood to the heart from the body tissues

e. Blood clot

f. Abnormal opening from one area to other area or to outside of the body

g. To go around

h. Surgically placed device that directs an electrical current shock to the heart to restore rhythm

11. _____ Artery

12. _____ Vein

13. _____ Aneurysm

14. _____ Embolism

15. _____ Thrombosis

16. _____ Endarterectomy

17. _____ Angioplasty

18. _____ Injection

19. _____ Catheter

20. _____ Arteriovenous fistula

21. _____ Anomaly

22. _____ Ischemia

23. _____ Cardiopulmonary bypass

24. _____ Fistula

25. _____ Shunt

i. Blockage of a blood vessel by a blood clot or other matter that has moved from another area of the body through the circulatory system

j. Direct communication (passage) between an artery and vein

k. Tube placed into the body to put fluid in or take fluid out

l. Surgical or percutaneous procedure on a vessel to dilate the vessel opening, used in treatment of atherosclerotic disease

m. Electrode of the pacemaker is placed only in the atrium or only in the ventricle, but not in both places

n. Membranous sac enclosing the heart and ends of the great vessels

o. Vessel that carries oxygenated blood from the heart to the body tissues

p. A sac of clotted blood of fluid formed in the circulatory system (e.g., vein or artery)

q. Incision into an artery to remove the inner lining to remove disease or blockage

r. Divert or make an artificial passage

s. Refers to the heart and lungs

t. Electrodes of the pacemaker are placed in both the atrium and the ventricle of the heart

u. Deficient blood supply caused by obstruction of the circulatory system

v. Chamber in the upper part of the heart

w. Electrical device that controls the beating of the heart by electrical impulses

x. Chamber in the lower part of the heart

y. Abnormality

26. The term that describes the procedure in which the surgeon withdraws fluid from the pericardial space by means of a needle inserted into the space is _____.

27. Codes for excision of cardiac tumors are divided based on whether the tumor is located _____ or _____.

28. What are the names of two devices that are inserted into the body to electrically shock the heart into regular rhythm?

    _____ and _____.

29. The two approaches used to insert devices that electrically shock the heart into regular rhythm are _____ and

    _____.

30. If the patient is returned to the operating room for repositioning or replacement of the pacemaker or cardioverter-defibrillator during the global period, modifier _____ would be appended to the code.

31. If a physician implanted a pacemaker and 10 days later the patient returns for removal of sutures, would you charge for the service?

    _____

32. If a patient is seen for a rash on the heel of the foot by the same physician who implanted a pacemaker 20 days earlier, would you bill for the office service for the rash? _____

33. When you bill for E/M services unrelated to a pacemaker implantation during the allowable follow-up days, what modifier would you use on the code to alert the third-party payer? _____

34. What are the four cardiac valves? _____,

    _____, _____, and _____.

35. What is the name of the device that can be surgically implanted into the subcutaneous tissue in the upper left quadrant with leads running outside the body to record heart rhythms when the patient depresses a button? _____

36. What arteries feed the heart? _____

37. When a heart artery is clogged and the heart muscle performs at a low level as a result of a lack of blood, the condition is called

    _____ _____ ischemia.

38. When the heart artery is clogged and the heart muscle dies, the condition is called _____ ischemia.

39. A mass of undissolved matter in the blood that is transported by the blood current is a _____.

40. Local anesthesia, catheter introduction, and injection of

    _____ _____ are procedures that are included in a vascular injection.

PRACTICAL

Using the CPT manual, code the following:

41. Valvuloplasty of the aortic valve using transventricular dilation with cardiopulmonary bypass.

    Code: _____

42. Replacement aortic valve, with cardiopulmonary bypass.

    Code: _____

43. Valvuloplasty, tricuspid valve, with ring insertion.

    Code: _____

44. Repair of a coronary arteriovenous fistula, without cardiopulmonary bypass.

    Code: _____

45. Routine ECG with 12 leads with both the professional and technical components.

    Code: _____

46. External electrical cardioversion.

    Code: _____

47. Percutaneous balloon angioplasty; one vessel.

    Code: _____

48. CPR (Cardiopulmonary resuscitation)

    Code: _____

49. Electrocardiogram with interpretation and report only.

    Code: _____

50. Bypass graft of the common carotid artery using synthetic vein.

    Code: _____

51. Ligation of temporal artery.

    Code: _____

52. Ligation of a common iliac vein.

    Code: _____

53. Open transluminal balloon angioplasty aortic artery.

    Code: _____

54. Coronary artery bypass, single artery.

    Code: _____

55. Coronary artery bypass four veins, no arteries.

    Code(s): _____

56. Repair of intraabdominal blood vessel with a vein graft.

    Code(s): _____

57. Insertion of a percutaneous intraaortic balloon assist device.

    Code(s): _____

58. Repair of a traumatic arteriovenous fistula of the extremity.

    Code(s): _____

59. Repair atrial septal defect, secundum, with bypass and patch.

    Code(s): _____

60. Repair of a patent ductus arteriosus by division on a 16-year-old patient.

    Code(s): _____

61. Reoperation of a one coronary bypass graft and one vein bypass graft.

    Code(s): _____.

REPORTS

Toward the end of this textbook, you will find a section titled Reports, which contains original reports. Read the reports indicated below and supply the appropriate CPT code(s) on the following lines:

62. Report 25 🌑 Code(s): _____

63. Report 26 🌑 Code(s): _____

64. Report 27 🌑 Code(s): _____

CHAPTER 8

Female Genital System and Maternity Care and Delivery

THEORY

Female Genital Terminology

Without the use of reference material, match the following terms to the correct definitions:

1. _____ Vulva

2. _____ Perineum

3. _____ Introitus

4. _____ Vagina

5. _____ Cervix uteri

6. _____ Corpus uteri

7. _____ Oviduct

8. _____ Salpingo-

9. _____ Oophor-

10. _____ Curettage

11. _____ Dilation

a. Herniation of the bladder into the vagina

b. Rounded, cone-shaped neck of the uterus, part of it protruding into the vagina

c. Prefix meaning ovary

d. External female genitalia, including labia majora, labia minora, clitoris, and vaginal opening

e. Uterus

f. Herniation of the rectal wall through the posterior wall of the vagina

g. Prefix meaning tube

h. Opening or entrance to the vagina from the uterus

i. Scraping of a cavity using a spoon-shaped instrument

12. _____ Cystocele   j.   Expansion

13. _____ Rectocele   k.   Area between the vulva and anus; also known as the pelvic floor

l.   Canal from the external female genitalia to the uterus

m.   Fallopian tube

Maternity Care and Delivery Terminology

Match the following terms to the correct definitions:

14. _____ Antepartum   a.   Turning of the fetus from a presentation other than cephalic (head down) to cephalic for ease of birth

15. _____ Postpartum

16. _____ Abortion   b.   Termination of pregnancy

17. _____ Delivery   c.   Surgical opening through abdominal wall for delivery

18. _____ Cesarean

d.   Before childbirth

19. _____ Ectopic

e.   After childbirth

20. _____ Version

f.   Pregnancy outside the uterus (e.g., in the fallopian tube)

21. _____ Amniocentesis

22. _____ Cordocentesis   g.   Childbirth

23. _____ Chorionic villus sampling (CVS)   h.   Incision into the uterus

i.   Surgical removal of the uterus

j.   Percutaneous aspiration of amniotic fluid

24. _____ Hysterotomy

k.   Surgical removal of ovary

25. _____ Salpingectomy

l.   Biopsy of the outermost part of the placenta

26. _____ Oophorectomy

27. _____ Hysterectomy   m.   Suturing of the uterus

28. _____ Hysterorrhaphy   n.   Repression of uterine contractions

29. _____ Tocolysis   o.   Surgical removal of a fallopian tube

30. _____ VBAC   p.   Vaginal delivery after previous cesarean delivery

q.   Procedure to obtain a fetal blood sample, also called a percutaneous umbilical blood sampling

Without the use of reference material, answer the following:

31. Plastic repair of the _____ is surgical repair of the opening of the vagina.

32. The cutting into the vagina to gain access to the pelvic cavity is

    _____.

33. The cutting into the vagina to gain access to a peritoneal cul de sac

    abscess is _____.

34. A vaginal support device is a _____.

35. When reporting the service of the introduction of a diaphragm, the cost of the diaphragm is included in the introduction.

    True _____ False _____

36. The term that describes the procedure in which the surgeon strengthens the wall of the weakened vagina by pulling together the weakened area with sutures.

    _____

37. The microscope that is used to view the vagina is a _____.

38. The services described in the Manipulation category of the Vagina

    subheading require this type of anesthesia. _____

39. LEEP means _____.

40. Endometrial _____ is a biopsy of the mucous lining of the uterus.

41. What one procedure represents the majority of the codes in the corpus

    uteri subheading? _____

42. The cost of an IUD is included in the code for the insertion.

    True _____ False _____

43. A hysterosalpingography would have a component code from what

    section of the CPT manual? _____

44. The first rule of a laparoscopy is that a surgical laparoscopy always

    includes a _____ laparoscopy.

45. In what subheading would you find the codes to report fallopian tube services?

   _____

46. The three methods of tubal ligation are ligation, _____,

   and _____.

47. Gestation is divided into three time periods called _____.

48. The first gestation time period is LMP to week _____, the

   second is week _____ to 27, and the third is week

   _____ to the EDC.

49. What does EDC stand for?

   _____ of _____.

50. Preparation of the cervix for birth or dilation is termed cervical

   _____.

51. If a physician other than the attending provided only one office visit to a patient before delivery, a code from what section of the CPT manual

   would be used to report this service? _____

52. The time after delivery is referred to as _____.

PRACTICAL

Using the CPT manual, code the following:

53. Dilation of the vagina under anesthesia.

    Code: _____

54. Plastic repair of a urethrocele.

    Code: _____

55. Labial adhesions lysis.

    Code: _____

56. Simple complete vulvectomy.

    Code(s): _____

57. Surgical hysteroscopy with polypectomy and dilatation and curettage.

    Code: _____

58. Transposition of the left ovary.

    Code: _____

59. Bilateral wedge resection of ovaries.

    Code: _____

60. Therapeutic amniocentesis with amniotic fluid reduction.

    Code: _____

61. Drainage of a cyst of the left ovary using the vaginal approach.

    Code(s): _____

62. Surgical treatment of a second trimester missed abortion.

    Code(s): _____

63. Cesarean delivery only.

    Code(s): _____

64. Hysterorrhaphy of a ruptured uterus.

    Code(s): _____

65. Fetal contraction stress tests, antepartum.

    Code(s): _____

66. Radical vaginal hysterectomy.

     Code(s): _____

67. Marsupialization of Bartholin's gland cyst.

     Code(s): _____

68. Excision of Bartholin's gland.

     Code(s): _____

69. Destruction of extensive vaginal lesions.

     Code(s): _____

REPORTS

Toward the end of this textbook, you will find a section titled Reports, which contains original reports. Code only the primary surgery. Read the report indicated below and supply the appropriate CPT code(s) on the following lines:

70. Report 20 Code(s): _____

71. Report 28 Code(s): _____

72. Report 29 Code(s): _____

73. Report 30 Code(s): _____

CHAPTER 9

General Surgery I

THEORY

Male Genital Terminology

Without the use of reference material, match the following terms to the correct definitions:

1. _____ Cavernosa-saphenous

2. _____ Orchiectomy

3. _____ Hydrocele

4. _____ Vasogram

5. _____ Varicocele

6. _____ Vas deferens

a. Tube that carries sperm from the epididymis to vein shunt the urethra

b. Swelling of a scrotal vein

c. Creation of a connection between the cavity of the penis and a vein

d. Castration

e. Sac of fluid

f. Recording of the flow in the vas deferens

Without reference material, match the following terms to the correct definitions:

7. _____ Electrodesiccation

8. _____ Corpora cavernosa

9. _____ Epididymis

10. _____ Cavernosography

11. _____ Cavernosometry

12. _____ Plethysmography

13. _____ Hypospadias

14. _____ Vesiculectomy

15. _____ Prostatotomy

a. Excision of a seminal vesicle

b. Determining the changes in volume of an organ part or body

c. Incision into the prostate

d. Destruction of a lesion by the use of electrical current radiated through a needle

e. A tube located on the top of the testes that stores sperm

f. Measurements of the pressure in a cavity (e.g., penis)

g. Two cavities of the penis

h. Radiographic measurement of a cavity (e.g., the main part of the penis)

i. Congenital deformity of the urethra in which the urethral opening is on the underside of the penis rather than on the end.

Without reference material, match the following terms to the correct definitions:

16. _____ Lymphadenectomy

17. _____ Priapism

18. _____ Chordee

19. _____ Urethroplasty

20. _____ Penoscrotal

21. _____ Spermatocele

a. Surgical repair of the urethra

b. Referring to the penis and scrotum

c. Painful condition in which the penis is constantly erect

d. Excision of lymph node(s)

e. Condition resulting in the penis being bent downward

f. Cyst filled with spermatozoa

Without reference material, match the following terms to the correct definitions:

22. _____ Tumescence

23. _____ Cavernosa-corpus spongiosum shunt

24. _____ Cavernosa-glans penis fistulization

a. Creation of a connection between a cavity of the penis and the urethra

b. Creation of a connection between a cavity of the penis and the glans penis, which overlaps the penis cavity

25. _____ Orchiopexy

26. _____ Vasovasostomy

27. _____ Vasovasorrhaphy

c. Reversal of a vasectomy

d. Surgical procedure to release undescended testis

e. Suturing of the vas deferens

f. State of being swollen

Without reference material, match the following terms to the correct definitions:

28. _____ Epididymectomy

29. _____ Epididymovasostomy

30. _____ Vasotomy

31. _____ Vesiculotomy

32. _____ Seminal vesicle

33. _____ Tunica vaginalis

a. Creation of a new connection between the vas deferens and epididymis

b. Creation of an opening in the vas deferens

c. Covering of the testes

d. Incision into the seminal vesicle

e. Glands that secrete fluid into the vas deferens

f. Surgical removal of the epididymis

Urinary System Terminology

Match the following terms to the correct definitions:

34. _____ Calculus/calculi

35. _____ Cystolithectomy

36. _____ Cystometrogram (CMG)

37. _____ Endopyelotomy

38. _____ Exstrophy

39. _____ Nephrectomy

40. _____ Fulguration

41. _____ Kock pouch

42. _____ Lithotripsy

43. _____ Marsupialization

a. Procedure of the bladder and ureters with insertion of a stent

b. Kidney removal

c. Crushing of a gallbladder or urinary bladder stone followed by irrigation to wash the fragment out

d. A concretion of mineral salts, also called a stone

e. Surgical creation of a urinary bladder from a segment of the ileum

f. Condition in which an organ is turned inside out

g. Measurement of the pressures and capacity of the urinary bladder

44. _____ Nephro-

45. _____ Nephrostomy

h. Creation of a channel into the renal pelvis of the kidney

i. Surgical procedure that creates an open pouch from an internal abscess

j. Removal of a calculus from the urinary bladder

k. Use of electrical current to destroy tissue

l. Prefix meaning kidney

Without reference material, match the following terms to the correct definitions:

46. _____ Perivesical

47. _____ Perirenal

48. _____ Pyelo-

49. _____ Pyeloplasty

50. _____ Pyelostomy

51. _____ Renal pelvis

52. _____ Retroperitoneal

53. _____ Transureteroureterostomy

54. _____ Ureterolithotomy

55. _____ Ureterotomy

56. _____ Urethrocystography

57. _____ Urethrorrhaphy

a. Prefix meaning renal pelvis

b. Removal of a stone from the ureter

c. Surgical connection of one ureter to the other ureter

d. Surgical creation of an opening into the renal pelvis

e. Suturing of the urethra

f. Behind the sac holding the abdominal organs and viscera (peritoneum)

g. Around the kidney

h. Radiography of the bladder and urethra

i. Around the bladder

j. Funnel-shaped sac in the kidney where urine is received

k. Surgical reconstruction of the renal pelvis

l. Incision into the ureter

Digestive Terminology

Match the following terms to the correct definitions:

58. _____ Gloss-

59. _____ Gastro-

60. _____ Anastomosis

61. _____ Hernia

62. _____ Gastrointestinal

63. _____ Ostomy

64. _____ Colostomy

65. _____ Ileostomy

66. _____ Jejunostomy

a. Artificial opening between the colon and the abdominal wall

b. Prefix meaning tongue

c. Organ or tissue protruding through the wall or cavity that usually contains it

d. Prefix meaning stomach

e. Artificial opening between the ileum and the abdominal wall

f. Surgical connection of two tubular structures, such as two pieces of the intestine

g. Pertaining to the stomach and intestine

h. Artificial opening

i. Artificial opening between the jejunum and the abdominal wall

Without reference material, match the following terms to the correct definitions:

67. _____ Gastrostomy

68. _____ Proctosigmoidoscopy

69. _____ Sigmoidoscopy

70. _____ Colonoscopy

71. _____ Cholangiography

72. _____ Chole-

73. _____ Hepa-

74. _____ Incarcerated

75. _____ Reducible

a. Regarding hernias, a constricted, irreducible hernia that may cause obstruction of an intestine

b. Artificial opening between the stomach and the abdominal wall

c. Radiographic recording of the bile ducts

d. Able to be corrected or put back into a normal position

e. Fiberscopic examination of the entire colon that may include part of the terminal ileum

f. Prefix meaning liver

g. Fiberscopic examination of the entire rectum and sigmoid colon that may include a portion of the descending colon

h. Prefix meaning bile

i. Fiberscopic examination of the sigmoid colon and rectum

Mediastinum and Diaphragm Terminology

Match the following terms to the correct definitions:

76. _____ Mediastinum

77. _____ Diaphragm

78. _____ Mediastinotomy

79. _____ Fundoplasty

80. _____ Pyloroplasty

81. _____ Diaphragmatic hernia

82. _____ Mediastinoscopy

83. _____ Imbrication

84. _____ Transthoracic

85. _____ Transabdominal

86. _____ Paraesophageal hiatus hernia

87. _____ Gastroplasty

88. _____ Vagotomy

a. Overlapping

b. Surgical separation of the vagus nerve

c. Muscular wall that separates the thoracic and abdominal cavities

d. Incision and repair of the pyloric channel

e. Operation on the stomach for repair or reconfiguration

f. Repair of the bottom of an organ or muscle

g. Hernia that is near the esophagus

h. Hernia of the diaphragm

i. Across the abdomen

j. Cutting into the mediastinum

k. Across the thorax

l. Use of an endoscope inserted through a small incision to view the mediastinum

m. That area between the lungs that contains the heart, aorta, trachea, lymph nodes, thymus gland, esophagus, and bronchial tubes

PRACTICAL

Using the CPT manual, code the following:

89. Endoscopy for resection of renal tumor through an established stoma.

    Code: _____

90. Aspiration of a renal cyst through percutaneous needle.

    Code: _____

91. Ureteroureterostomy.

    Code: _____

92. Transurethral incision of the prostate.

    Code: _____

93. Uvulectomy.

    Code: _____

94. Ligation of an intraoral salivary duct.

    Code: _____

95. Transection of esophagus with repair of esophageal varices.

    Code: _____

96. Enterotomy of the small intestine for removal of a foreign body.

    Code: _____

97. Complicated revision of a colostomy.

    Code: _____

98. Frenotomy, labial.

    Code: _____

99. Excision of a palate lesion without closure.

    Code: _____

100. Removal of a foreign body from the pharynx.

    Code: _____

101. Amy is an 18-year-old with severe snoring. She is having an adenoidectomy done in order to treat this.

    Code: _____

102. Partial colectomy with colostomy.

    Code: _____

103. Repair of an incarcerated recurrent inguinal hernia.

    Code: _____

104. Excision of a mediastinal cyst.

    Code: _____

105. Transthoracic repair of a diaphragmatic hernia.

    Code: _____

106. Cystourethroscopy.

    Code: _____

107. Abdominal orchiopexy to release intraabdominal testes.

    Code: _____

108. Complicated prostatomy of a prostate cyst.

    Code: _____

109. Full thickness repair of the vermilion of the lip.

    Code(s): _____

110. Simple repair of 1.6-cm laceration of floor of mouth.

    Code(s): _____

111. Bilateral parotid duct diversion.

    Code(s): _____

112. Esophagogastric fundoplasty.

    Code(s): _____

113. Biopsy of the stomach by laparotomy.

    Code(s): _____

114. Nontube ileostomy.

    Code(s): _____

115. Colorrhaphy for multiple perforations of large intestine sustained in auto accident.

    Code(s): _____

116. Incision and drainage of perirectal abscess.

        Code(s): _____

117. Diagnostic abdominal laparoscopy.

        Code(s): _____

118. Closure of nephrocutaneous fistula.

        Code(s): _____

119. A steroid injection for urethral stricture using a cystourethroscope.

        Code(s): _____

120. Total urethrectomy of a 44-year-old male.

        Code(s): _____

121. Circumcision using clamp.

        Code(s): _____

122. Excision of Skene's glands.

        Code(s): _____

123. Bilateral shunt of corpora cavernosa–saphenous vein for priapism.

        Code(s): _____

124. Vasovasorrhaphy.

        Code(s): _____

125. Exposure of the prostate for insertion of radioactive substance.

        Code(s): _____

126. Surgical reduction of torsion of testis with fixation of contralateral testis.

        Code(s): _____

127. Distal hypospadias repair with chordee using a V-flap advancement, completed in one stage.

        Code(s): _____

128. Simple destruction of four lesions of the penis using cryosurgery.

        Code(s): _____

129. Repair of an incomplete circumcision.

        Code(s): _____

130. Drainage of a scrotal wall abscess.

    Code(s): _____

131. Ureterectomy, with repair of the bladder cuff.

    Code(s): _____

REPORTS

Toward the end of this textbook, you will find a section titled Reports, which contains original reports. Read the reports indicated below and supply the appropriate CPT codes on the following lines:

132. Report 22 🐾 Code(s): _____

133. Report 31 🐾 Code(s): _____

134. Report 32 🐾 Code(s): _____

135. Report 33 🐾 Code(s): _____

136. Report 34 🐾 Code(s): _____

137. Report 35 🐾 Code(s): _____

138. Report 36 🐾 Code(s): _____

139. Report 37 🐾 Code(s): _____

140. Report 38 🐾 Code(s): _____

141. Report 39 🐾 Code(s): _____

142. Report 81 🐾 Code(s): _____

143. Report 82 🐾 Code(s): _____

144. Report 83 🐾 Code(s): _____

145. Report 84 🐾 Code(s): _____

CHAPTER 10

General Surgery II

THEORY

Hemic and Lymphatic Terminology

Without the use of reference material, match the following terms to the correct definition:

1. _____ Axillary nodes

2. _____ Splenectomy

3. _____ Splenoportography

4. _____ Allogenic

5. _____ Autologous, autogenous

6. _____ Aspiration

7. _____ Stem cell

8. _____ Transplantation

9. _____ Lymph node

10. _____ Lymphadenitis

a. Behind the sac holding the abdominal organs and viscera (peritoneum)

b. Grafting of tissue from one source to another

c. Excision of the spleen

d. Immature blood cells

e. Incision into a lymphatic vessel

f. Insertion of a tube into a duct or cavity

g. Lymph nodes located next to the large vein in the neck

h. Radiographic procedure to allow visualization of the splenic and portal veins of the spleen

11. _____ Lymphangiotomy
12. _____ Thoracic duct
13. _____ Lymphadenectomy
14. _____ Retroperitoneal
15. _____ Jugular nodes
16. _____ Cystic hygroma
17. _____ Cloquet's node
18. _____ Inguinofemoral
19. _____ Cannulation
20. _____ Abscess

i. Of the same species, but genetically different

j. Inflammation of a lymph node

k. Collection and distribution point for lymph and the largest lymph vessel located in the chest

l. Excision of a lymph node (or nodes)

m. From oneself

n. Congenital deformity of benign tumor of the lymphatic system

o. Also called a gland; it is the highest of the deep groin lymph nodes

p. Use of a needle and syringe to withdraw fluid

q. Station along the lymphatic system

r. Term that refers to the groin and thigh

s. Lymph nodes located in the armpit

t. Localization of pus

Endocrine System Terminology

Match the following terms to the correct definitions:

21. _____ Isthmus
22. _____ Isthmus, thyroid
23. _____ Isthmusectomy
24. _____ Contralateral
25. _____ Thyroidectomy
26. _____ Thyroglossal duct
27. _____ Thymectomy
28. _____ Adrenal
29. _____ Thyroid
30. _____ Thymus

a. Glands located on the top of the kidneys that produce steroid hormones

b. Produces a hormone to mobilize calcium from the bones to the blood

c. Connection of two regions or structures

d. Surgical removal of the thyroid

e. Produces hormones important to the immune response

f. Surgical removal of the isthmus

g. Surgical removal of the thymus

h. Part of the endocrine system that produces hormones that regulate metabolism

31. _____ Parathyroid

   i. Tissue connection between right and left thyroid lobes

   j. Connection of the thyroid and the pharynx and continuation with the endocrinal floor of the mouth

   k. Affecting the opposite side

Nervous System Terminology

Match the following terms to the correct definitions:

32. _____ Cranium

33. _____ Skull

34. _____ Stereotaxis

35. _____ Laminectomy

36. _____ Somatic Nerve

37. _____ Sympathetic nerve

38. _____ Peripheral nerves

39. _____ Shunt

40. _____ Central nervous system

   a. A method of identifying a specific area or point in the brain

   b. Part of the peripheral nervous system that controls automatic body function and sympathetic nerves activated under stress

   c. That part of the skeleton that encloses the brain

   d. Divert or make an artificial passage

   e. Twelve pairs of cranial nerves, 31 pairs of spinal nerves, and autonomic nervous system; connects peripheral receptors to the brain and spinal cord

   f. Sensory or motor nerve

   g. Entire skeletal framework of the head

   h. Surgical excision of the lamina

   i. Brain and spinal cord

Eye and Ocular Adnexa Terminology

Match the following terms to the correct definitions:

41. _____ Keratoplasty

42. _____ Evisceration

43. _____ Enucleation

44. _____ Exenteration

45. _____ Cataract

46. _____ Sclera

   a. Prefix meaning eye

   b. Prefix meaning tear/tear duct

   c. Surgical repair of the cornea

   d. Removal of an organ (eye)

   e. Opaque covering on or in the lens

   f. Those parts of the eye behind the lens

47. _____ Conjunctiva

48. _____ Uveal

49. _____ Tarsorrhaphy

50. _____ Ocular adnexa

51. _____ Anterior segment

52. _____ Posterior segment

53. _____ Blephar/o-

54. _____ Cor/o-

55. _____ Cyclo/o-

56. _____ Dacry/o-

57. _____ Kerat/o-

58. _____ Ocul/o-

59. _____ Dacryocyst/o-

60. _____ Vitre/o-

61. _____ Astigmatism

62. _____ Strabismus

g. Lining of the eyelids and covering of the sclera

h. Removal of an organ all in one piece

i. Pulling the viscera outside the body through an incision

j. White outer portion of the eyeball

k. Vascular tissue of the choroids, ciliary body, and iris

l. Prefix meaning cornea

m. Prefix meaning pertaining to the vitreous body of the eye

n. Prefix meaning ciliary body or eye muscle

o. Suturing together of the eyelids

p. Those parts of the eye in the front of and including the lens, orbit, extraocular muscles, and eyelid

q. Orbit, extraocular muscles, and eyelid

r. Prefix meaning pertaining to the lacrimal sac

s. Extraocular muscle deviation resulting in unequal visual axes

t. Condition in which the refractive surfaces of the eyes are unequal

u. Prefix meaning eyelid

v. Prefix meaning pupil

Auditory System Terminology

Match the following terms to the correct definitions:

63. _____ Aural atresia

64. _____ Transmastoid antrostomy

65. _____ Labyrinth

66. _____ Tympanic neurectomy

67. _____ Fenestration

68. _____ Parts of the external ear

69. _____ Parts of the middle ear

70. _____ Parts of the inner ear

71. _____ Mastoid-

72. _____ Myring-

73. _____ Audi-

74. _____ Exostosis

75. _____ Oto-

76. _____ Salping(o)-

77. _____ Apicectomy

a. Prefix meaning hearing

b. Auricle, pinna, external acoustic, and meatus

c. Prefix meaning ear

d. Prefix meaning (eustachian) tube

e. Vestibule, semicircular canals, and cochlea

f. Excision of the tympanic nerve

g. Congenital absence of the external auditory canal

h. Creation of a new opening (e.g., on the inner wall of the middle ear)

i. Malleus, incus, and stapes

j. A bony growth

k. Prefix meaning posterior temporal bone

l. Excision of a portion of the temporal bone

m. Called a simple mastoidectomy, it creates an opening in the mastoid for drainage

n. Inner connecting cavities, such as the internal ear

o. Prefix meaning eardrum

PRACTICAL

Using the CPT manual, code the following:

78. Injection procedure for identification of the sentinel node.

    Code: _____

79. Radical cervical lymphadenectomy, unilateral.

    Code: _____

80. Drainage of an extensive lymph node abscess.

    Code: _____

81. Autologous bone marrow transplant.

    Code: _____

82. Incision and drainage of an infected thyroglossal duct cyst.

    Code(s): _____

83. Removal of a complete cerebrospinal fluid shunt system; without replacement.

    Code(s): _____

84. Suture of the posterior tibial nerve.

    Code(s): _____

85. Incision and drainage of conjunctival cysts of left and right eyes.

    Code(s): _____

86. Optic nerve decompression of the right eye.

    Code(s): _____

87. Removal of a embedded foreign body of the eyelid.

    Code(s): _____

88. Myringoplasty of the left ear.

    Code(s): _____

89. Single stage reconstruction of the external auditory canal for congenital atresia.

    Code(s): _____

90. Stapedectomy with footplate drill out.

    🔗 Code(s): _____

91. Excision of a lacrimal sac.

    🔗 Code(s): _____

REPORTS

Toward the end of this textbook, you will find a section titled Reports, which contains original reports. Read the reports indicated below and supply the appropriate CPT codes on the following lines:

92. Report 40   Code(s): _____

93. Report 41   Code(s): _____

94. Report 42   Code(s): _____

95. Report 43   Code(s): _____

96. Report 44   Code(s): _____

97. Report 85   Code(s): _____

98. Report 86   Code(s): _____

99. Report 87   Code(s): _____

100. Report 88   Code(s): _____

CHAPTER 11

—

Radiology Section

THEORY

Match the following terms to the correct definition:

1. _____ Anterior (ventral)   a. Toward the midline of the body

2. _____ Posterior (dorsal)   b. Toward the head or the upper part of the
body; also known as cephalad or cephalic

3. _____ Superior

   c. In front of
4. _____ Inferior

   d. Away from the midline of the body (to
5. _____ Medial   the side)

6. _____ Lateral   e. In back of

   f. Away from the head or the lower part of
the body; also known as caudad or caudal

Match the following radiographic procedures to the correct structures imaged:

7. _____ Fluoroscopy   a. Radiographic contrast medium

8. _____ Magnetic resonance   b. Procedure for viewing the interior
imaging (MRI)   of the body using x-rays and
projecting the image onto a
9. _____ Tomography   television screen

10. _____ Xeroradiography   c. Photoelectric process of radiographs

11. _____ Barium

12. _____ Biometry

d. Application of a statistical method to a biological fact

e. Procedure that uses nonionizing radiation to view the body in a cross-sectional view

f. Procedure that allows viewing of a single plane of the body by blurring out all but that particular level

Match the following radiographic procedures to the correct structures imaged:

13. _____ Arthrography

14. _____ Cholangiography

15. _____ Cystography

16. _____ Diskography

17. _____ Epididymography

18. _____ Hysterosalpingography

19. _____ Lymphangiography

20. _____ Myelography

21. _____ Urography

22. _____ Venography

a. Uterine cavity and fallopian tubes

b. Intervertebral joint

c. Kidneys, renal pelvis, ureters, and bladder

d. Bile ducts

e. Joint

f. Veins and tributaries

g. Subarachnoid space of the spine

h. Epididymis

i. Urinary bladder

j. Lymphatic vessels and nodes

PRACTICAL

Using the CPT manual, answer the following:

23. What is the unlisted diagnostic nuclear medicine code used for cardiovascular procedures? _____

24. What is the add on code for coronary intravascular brachytherapy?

    _____

25. The modifier used to indicate the professional component only is

    _____

26. What modifier is used to indicate a technical component?

    _____

27. Supervision and interpretation of angiography, spinal, selective.

    Code: _____

28. Radiological examination of the eye for foreign body.

    Code: _____

29. Radiological examination of mastoids, four views per side.

    Code: _____

30. Radiological examination of the ribs, two views.

    Code: _____

31. MRI of the neck, with contrast material.

    Code: _____

32. Computed tomography of the thoracic spine, without contrast.

    Code: _____

33. Complete hip x-ray study, two views.

    Code: _____

34. Complete four-view radiological examination of the wrist.

    Code: _____

35. Supervision and interpretation of transluminal atherectomy, renal.

    Code(s): _____

36. An established patient is seen in the office complaining of severe headaches. To diagnose and treat the patient, the physician needs to identify a cause for these headaches. He performs an expanded problem-focused history and examination and orders a CT scan of the head. Contrast was used.

    🐾 Code(s): _____

37. A new patient is admitted to the hospital on an observation status after a fall at home. A comprehensive history is collected and a general, multisystem comprehensive physical examination is performed. After talking to the patient and relatives and performing the examination, the physician finds that the patient has a number of symptoms that are usually due to an increase in intracranial pressure. The physician considers this patient's problems to be of moderately severe complexity. The MDM complexity is moderate. A CT scan of the brain is done. Brain lesions are discovered, and the physician advises radiation therapy. The patient is sent to the clinic's radiology department, where an A-scan ophthalmic biometry by ultrasound is done. The patient has therapeutic radiology treatment planning that is simple. Later the patient has radiation treatment delivery to a single area up to 5 MeV. The patient continues with weekly radiology therapy management, five treatments.

    🐾 Code(s): _____

38. A new patient is seen in the clinic for an office consult. The patient has a mass in the neck with related pain and dysphagia. The consulting physician performs an expanded problem-focused history and examination, and low-complexity decision making. A CT scan of the patient's neck is ordered. This was done with and without contrast.

    🐾 Code(s): _____

39. A patient was admitted to the hospital for removal of a pericardial clot. The physician orders a real time chest ultrasound. Chest magnetic resonance (proton) imaging is also ordered (without contrast). A pericardiotomy is performed for removal of clot.

    🐾 Code(s): _____

40. Radiological examination, ankle, two views.

    🐾 Code(s): _____

41. X-ray of a 6-month-old's arm; 2 views.

    🐾 Code(s): _____

42. Unilateral selective pulmonary angiography, supervision and interpretation.

    🐾 Code(s): _____

43. Fluoroscopic guidance for needle placement.

    🐾 Code(s): _____

44. Computed tomography guidance for stereotactic localization.

    Code(s): _____

45. Transrectal ultrasound.

    Code(s): _____

46. Four-view x-ray of the lumbosacral spine.

    Code(s): _____

47. Myelography, cervical, radiological supervision and interpretation.

    Code(s): _____

48. Bilateral screening mammography.

    Code(s): _____

49. X-ray of the facial bones, 2 views.

    Code(s): _____

50. TMJ x-ray with mouth open and closed on one side of the mouth.

    Code(s): _____

51. X-ray of abdomen, single anteroposterior, and additional oblique and cone views.

    Code(s): _____

52. Percutaneous placement of gastrostomy tube, radiological supervision, and interpretation.

    Code(s): _____

53. Venography, superior sagittal sinus, radiological supervision and interpretation.

    Code(s): _____

54. Magnetic resonance spectroscopy.

    Code(s): _____

55. Intravascular ultrasound of a noncoronary vessel, radiological supervision and interpretation.

    Code(s): _____

56. Venography of unilateral extremity; radiological supervision and interpretation.

    Code(s): _____

REPORTS

Toward the end of this textbook, you will find a section titled Reports, which contains original reports. Read the reports indicated below and supply the appropriate CPT codes on the following lines:

57. Report 45 🐾   Code(s): _____

58. Report 46 🐾   Code(s): _____

59. Report 47 🐾   Code(s): _____

60. Report 48 🐾   Code(s): _____

61. Report 49 🐾   Code(s): _____

62. Report 50 🐾   Code(s): _____

63. Report 51 🐾   Code(s): _____

64. Report 52 🐾   Code(s): _____

65. Report 53 🐾   Code(s): _____

CHAPTER 12

—

Pathology/Laboratory Section

THEORY

Without the use of reference materials, answer the following:

1. In what section of the CPT manual will you find the codes to indicate the service of venipuncture?

   _____

2. When a laboratory drug test is qualitative it measures the

   _____ of the drug.

3. When a laboratory drug test is quantitative, it measures the

   _____ and the _____ of the drug.

4. When coding an evocative/suppression test, you may have an E/M code to indicate a prolonged period of time the physician spends with the patient during the testing process or a report of the injection or infusion service. What other service may you need to report?

   _____

5. A sample of tissue from a suspect area that is examined by a pathologist is a specimen, a block is a frozen piece of the specimen, and a _____ is a slice of the frozen block.

6. How many levels of surgical pathology are there? _____

7. If one breast specimen is received for pathological analysis and the pathologist examines two blocks of the specimen, how many codes would be used to report the service of analysis? _____

PRACTICAL

Using the CPT manual, code the following:

8. CARDIAC ENZYMES

Ref	Range	Units	12/18/XX
CPK	35-232 IU	69	0.0123
CKMB	0-10	ng/ml	1

CARDIAC MARKERS
12/18/XX   +123 TROPONIN I   <0.3 ng/ml

Troponin I Interpretation

≤0.4 ng/ml for apparently healthy individual

0.5–1.9 ng/ml for clinically Dx non-AMI patients

≥2.0 g/ml reasonably specific for AMI

Code(s): CPK, total: _____

CKMB (creatine kinase, cardiac fraction): _____

Troponin, quantitative: _____

9. GENERAL BLOOD CHEMISTRY

	Ref Range	Units	10/30/xx 0620	10/27/xx 1855
BUN	7-22	mg/dl		H 37
Sodium	136-145	mmol/L		138
Potassium	3.6-5.5	mmol/L		4.5
Creatinine	0.6-1.3	mg/dl	H 1.9	H 2.4
Uric acid	2.6-6.0	mg/dl	H 9.6	

Code(s): BUN:

Sodium: _____

Potassium: _____

Creatinine: _____

Uric acid: _____

10. An 84-year-old evaluated for renal failure, anemia, and hypertension.

Labs include

Magnesium: _____

Iron: _____

Phosphorus: _____

Total protein serum: _____

11. A 48-year-old female patient with hyperlipidemia, currently on Lipitor.

   Labs include:

   Hepatic function: _____

   Lipid panel: _____

12. A 20-year-old male in for labs due to chronic asthma.

   Labs include:

   Theophylline: _____

13. A 55-year-old male in for labs, digoxin level for his atrial fibrillation.

   Labs include:

   Digoxin: _____

REPORTS

Toward the end of this textbook, you will find a section titled Reports, which contains original reports. Read the reports indicated below and supply the appropriate CPT codes on the following lines:

14. Report 54 🐾 Code(s): _____

15. Report 55 🐾 Code(s): _____

16. Report 56 🐾 Code(s): _____

17. Report 57 🐾 Code(s): _____

18. Report 58 🐾 Code(s): _____

19. Report 59 🐾 Code(s): _____

20. Report 60 🐾 Code(s): _____

21. Report 61 🐾 Code(s): _____

22. Report 62 🐾 Code(s): _____

23. Report 63 🐾 Code(s): _____

24. Report 64 🐾 Code(s): _____

25. Report 65 🐾 Code(s): _____

26. Report 66 🐾 Code(s): _____

27. Report 67 🐾 Code(s): _____

CHAPTER 13

—

Medicine Section and Level II National Codes

THEORY

Without the use of reference material, match the following terms to the correct definitions:

1. _____ Aphakia

2. _____ Echography

3. _____ Gonioscopy

4. _____ Hemodialysis

5. _____ Modality

6. _____ Nystagmus

7. _____ Optokinetic

8. _____ Percutaneous

9. _____ Phlebotomy

10. _____ Retrograde

11. _____ Subcutaneous

12. _____ Tonometry

13. _____ Transcutaneous

a. Entering by way of the skin

b. Moving backward or against the usual direction of flow

c. Through the skin

d. Cleansing of the blood outside the body

e. Procedure for evaluation of inner ear disorders

f. Rapid involuntary eye movements

g. Cutting into a vein

h. Use of a scope to examine the angles of the eye

i. Movement of the eye to objects moving in the visual field

j. Ultrasound procedure in which sound waves are bounced off an internal organ and the resulting image is recorded

14. _____ Tympanometry

    k. Measurement of pressure or tension

    l. Tissue below dermis, primarily fat cells that insulate the body

    m. Absence of the lens of the eye

    n. Treatment method

Match the following administration methods for drugs:

15. _____ OTH   a. Subcutaneous

16. _____ IT   b. Inhalant solution

17. _____ IV   c. Various routes

18. _____ IM   d. Intrathecal

19. _____ SC   e. Intramuscular

20. _____ INH   f. Intravenous

21. _____ VAR   g. Other routes

Define the following terms:

22. Oscillating _____

23. Audiometry _____

24. Tympanometry _____

25. Electrocochleography _____

26. Orthoptic _____

27. Angioscopy _____

28. Electroretinography _____

29. Anomaloscope _____

30. Aphakia _____

31. Corneosclera _____

32. What are the three levels (level number and name) of HCPCS?

    a. _____

    b. _____

    c. _____

33. What are the K, G, Q, and S codes used for in the national codes?

_____

_____

34. Can you code directly from the national codes manual index?

Yes _____ No _____

35. Is there only one entry in the index of the national codes manual for each item?

Yes _____ No _____

36. In what section of the national codes manual would you locate the generic name of drugs?

_____

37. What are J Codes? _____

38. Under what route of administration would suppositories or catheter injections be classified? _____

39. What does the abbreviation DME stand for? _____

_____ _____

PRACTICAL

Using the CPT manual, code the following:

40. Three injections of allergy, providing extract and professional service.

    Code: _____

41. Two photo patch tests.

    Code(s): _____

42. Replacement of contact lenses.

    Code: _____

43. Patient is fitted for bifocal spectacles.

    Code: _____

44. Electrooculography with interpretation and report.

    Code: _____

45. Optokinetic nystagmus test.

    Code: _____

46. Positional nystagmus test, five positions.

    Code: _____

47. An esophagus acid reflux test with nasal catheter electrode placement for detection of gastroesophageal reflux.

    Code: _____

48. Peritoneal dialysis with two physician evaluations.

    Code: _____

49. Hypnotherapy.

    Code: _____

50. Bernstein test for esophagitis.

    Code: _____

51. Evaluation of auditory rehabilitation status, 1 hour.

    Code: _____

52. Family psychotherapy without the patient present.

    Code: _____

53. Hemodialysis access flow study to determine blood flow in grafts.

    Code: _____

54. Puretone audiometry; air and bone.

    Code: _____

55. Insertion of a Swan-Ganz catheter.

    Code: _____

56. Electronic analysis of a single chamber AICD, with reprogramming.

    🔾 Code(s): _____

57. Ventilation management for assist of breathing; second day for a hospital inpatient.

    🔾 Code(s): _____

58. Training for a prosthetic arm, 45 minutes.

    🔾 Code(s): _____

59. Oral conscious sedation provided by the same physician performing the diagnostic test on a 40-year-old patient for 30 minutes.

    🔾 Code(s): _____

60. GI tract intraluminal imaging.

    🔾 Code(s): _____

61. Administration of two vaccines.

    🔾 Code(s): _____

Each of the following questions has a HCPCS/National Level II code(s) in the answer. If you do not have a coding text for Level II codes, identify the item(s) that would be coded with a Level II code(s). Also, code E/M in addition to all medical and surgical services.

62. A 14-year-old boy is leaving the hospital after an open surgical repair of a left proximal fibula fracture. The patient needs a set of crutches because he is not allowed to bear any weight on his left leg. A prescription was ordered for a pair of forearm crutches.

    Code: _____ open repair of knee fracture

    HCPCS Item(s)/Code: _____

63. A 50-year-old female established patient has an excision of a 1.2-cm, benign skin lesion on her back, performed in the office. A surgical tray is used during the procedure.

    Code: _____

    HCPCS Item(s)/Code: _____

64. The patient is a 5-year-old female that was born severely premature. The patient had asthma develop with increasing progression and severity of the attacks. The patient is seen in the clinic for yet again another attack. The physician performs a detailed history, a problem-focused examination and moderate-complexity decision making. Decision is made to prescribe a nebulizer for home use. A portable nebulizer is prescribed.

    Code(s): _____

    HCPCS Item(s)/Code: _____

65. A 42-year-old male who was in a car accident 2 years ago is a paraplegic. He was admitted to the hospital 2 days ago with a UTI and today the physician was asked to consult regarding the decubitus ulcers. The patient has two fairly deep ulcers on his left buttock. An expanded problem history and examination was performed. Straightforward decision making was made. A prescription for a water pressure pad was ordered for the patient to take home from the hospital when discharged.

    Code(s): _____

    HCPCS Item(s)/Code: _____

66. An established patient with coronary artery disease is seen in his physician's office for an arthrocentesis with a 4-mg betamethasone sodium phosphate injection if the left knee.

    Code: _____

    HCPCS Item(s)/Code: _____

REPORTS

Toward the end of this textbook, you will find a section titled Reports, which contains original reports. Read the reports indicated below and supply the appropriate CPT codes on the following lines:

67. Report 68 🐾 Code(s): _____

68. Report 69 🐾 Code(s): _____

69. Report 70 🐾 Code(s): _____

70. Report 71 🐾 Code(s): _____

71. Report 72 🐾 Code(s): _____

72. Report 73 🐾 Code(s): _____

73. Report 74 🐾 Code(s): _____

74. Report 75 🐾 Code(s): _____

75. Report 76 🐾 Code(s): _____

76. Report 77 🐾 Code(s): _____

77. Report 78 🐾 Code(s): _____

78. Report 79 🐾 Code(s): _____

79. Report 80 🐾 Code(s): _____

CHAPTER 14

—

An Overview of the ICD-9-CM

THEORY

Without the use of reference material, answer the following:

1. E codes are located in Section:

   a. 3

   b. 2

   c. 1

   d. 0

2. Benign, malignant, and carcinoma in situ are examples of types of:

   a. Secondary sites

   b. Neoplasm behavior

   c. Borderline malignancy

   d. Primary sites

Match the abbreviations, punctuation, symbols, words, or typeface to the correct descriptions:

3. _____ [ ]

4. _____ NOS

5. _____ :

6. _____ §

7. _____ Italics

8. _____ Excludes

9. _____ Includes

10. _____ }

11. _____ NEC

12. _____ ( )

13. _____ *[ ]*

14. _____ Bold type

a. Incomplete term that needs one of the modifiers to make a code assignable

b. Used in Volume 2 to enclose the disease and procedure codes that are recorded with the code they are listed with

c. Typeface used for all codes and titles in Volume 1

d. Information is not available to code to a more specific category

e. Encloses a series of terms that are modified by the statement to the right

f. Encloses synonyms, alternative words, or explanatory phrases

g. Equals unspecified

h. Typeface used for all exclusion notes

i. Footnote or section mark

j. Appears under a three-digit code title to further define or explain category content

k. Encloses supplementary words and does not affect the code

l. Indicates terms that are to be coded elsewhere

Match the convention to the definition:

15. _____ See category

16. _____ Modifiers

17. _____ *See*

18. _____ Notes

19. _____ Subterms

20. _____ *See also*

21. _____ Eponym

a. Indented under main term and are essential to code selection

b. Terms in parentheses that are nonessential

c. Explicit direction to look elsewhere

d. Follows terms to define and give instructions

e. Directs coder to look under another term since all information is not under the first term

f. Directs coder to Volume 1

g. Disease/syndrome named for a person

Circle the correct answer for each of the following:

22. Volume 3 is primarily used by which of the following?

    a. Clinics

    b. Ambulatory centers

    c. Hospitals

    d. Nursing homes

23. Volume 3 is used to code what type of procedures?

    a. Surgical

    b. Therapeutic

    c. Diagnostic

    d. All of the above

Identify if the following statements are True or False:

24. The location of the Includes and Excludes notes has no bearing on the code selection. _____

25. Use of fourth and fifth digits, if available, is mandatory.

    _____

26. If the same condition is listed as both acute and chronic, the chronic condition is sequenced first._____

27. Four-digit codes are referred to as subcategory codes in Volume 1.

    _____

28. In Volume 2, Alphabetic Index, when the main term is modified by terms listed in parentheses following the main term, these modifiers are considered essential for code selection. _____

Underline the main term in the following:

29. Grief reaction

30. Fracture radius and ulna

31. Bowel obstruction

32. Erb's palsy

33. Supervision of high-risk pregnancy

34. Aortic stenosis

35. Rapid respiration

36. Actinomycosis meningitis

Identify as category, subcategory, and subclassification:

37. 066.1 _____

38. 070.43 _____

39. 220 _____

40. 274.11 _____

41. 284.9 _____

42. 337.21 _____

Are the following codes procedure codes or diagnosis codes?

43. 214.0 _____

44. 251.0 _____

45. 31.41 _____

46. 37.96 _____

47. 663.61 _____

CHAPTER 15

Using the ICD-9-CM

PRACTICAL

Using the ICD-9-CM, code the following:

1. Family history of gout.

   Code: _____

2. Encounter for cast removal.

   Code: _____

3. Encounter for vision examination.

   Code: _____

4. Status post cardiac pacemaker placement.

   Code: _____

5. Screening for yellow fever.

   Code: _____

6. Screening for malignant neoplasm of the colon.

   Code: _____

7. Observation for an alleged suicide attempt.

   Code: _____

8. Personal history of an allergy to latex.

   Code: _____

9. Vaccination for smallpox.

   Code: _____

10. Severe mental retardation due to previous viral encephalitis.

    Residual _____ Code: _____

    Cause _____ Code: _____

11. Nonunion of left tibia fracture (closed).

    Residual nonunion fracture. Code: _____

    Cause fracture, tibia. Code: _____

12. Osteoporosis due to previous poliomyelitis.

    Residual osteoporosis. Code: _____

    Cause poliomyelitis. Code: _____

13. Flaccid hemiplegia affecting dominant side due to cerebrovascular accident 4 months ago. Residual and cause flaccid hemiplegia, dominant side, CVA.

    Code: _____

14. Chronic hepatitis C.

    Code: _____

15. Tinea pedis.

    Code: _____

16. Mycobacterium pulmonary infection.

    Code: _____

17. Acute prostatitis due to streptococcus.

    Code(s): _____ _____

18. Hypokalemic syndrome.

    Code: _____

19. Adjustment of a colostomy tube for fitting.

    Code: _____

20. Malignant neoplasm of the tail of the pancreas.

    Code: _____

21. Screening for unspecified immunity disorder.

    Code: _____

22. Infection due to group B streptococcus.

    Code: _____

23. Mixed hyperlipidemia.

    Code: _____

24. Immunoglobulin G deficiency.

    Code: _____

25. Tumor abdomen.

    Code: _____

    M Code: _____

26. Diabetic retinopathy, type II, controlled.

    Code(s): _____ _____

27. Hepatocellular adenoma.

    Code: _____

    M Code: _____

28. Vitamin B_{12} deficiency.

    Code: _____

29. Gangrene, left great toe, due to diabetes mellitus, type I.

    Code(s): _____ _____

30. Vitamin D-resistant rickets.

    Code(s): _____

31. Unspecified thrombocytopenia.

    Code: _____

32. Wermer's syndrome.

    Code: _____

33. Active state of childhood autism.

    Code: _____

34. Screening for cystic fibrosis.

    Code: _____

35. Atypical bipolar affective disorder.

    Code: _____

36. Chronic lymphadenitis.

    Code: _____

37. Streptococcal septicemia.

    Code: _____

38. Toxic shock syndrome.

    Code: _____

39. Chronic schizophrenia, paranoid type.

    Code: _____

40. Carpal tunnel syndrome.

    Code: _____

41. Tobacco abuse.

    Code: _____

42. Pneumococcal meningitis.

    Code: _____

43. Panic attack, without agoraphobia.

    Code: _____

44. Parkinson's disease.

    Code: _____

45. Peripheral retinal edema.

    Code: _____

46. Meniere's disease in remission.

    Code: _____

47. Total traumatic cataract.

    Code: _____

48. Chronic follicular conjunctivitis.

    Code: _____

49. Sensorineural hearing loss.

    Code: _____

50. Malignant hypertensive heart disease, with heart failure.

    Code: _____

51. A 62-year-old male admitted to the hospital with acute subendocardial myocardial infarction.

    Code: _____

52. Arteriosclerotic cardiovascular disease.

    Code(s): _____ _____

53. Primary pulmonary hypertension.

    Code: _____

54. Fibrosis of the pericardium.

    Code: _____

55. Paroxysmal supraventricular tachycardia.

    Code: _____

56. Chronic diastolic heart failure.

    Code: _____

57. Stenosis of the renal arteries.

    Code: _____

58. Saddle embolus.

    Code: _____

59. Chronic lymphangitis.

    Code: _____

60. Acute frontal sinusitis.

    Code: _____

61. Abscess of the vocal cords.

    Code: _____

62. Chronic tonsillitis and adenoiditis.

    Code: _____

63. Acute exacerbation of chronic obstructive bronchitis.

    Code: _____

64. Abscess of the lung.

    Code: _____

65. Aphthous stomatitis.

    Code: _____

66. Chronic gastric ulcer with perforation.

    Code: _____

67. Hiatal hernia with obstruction.

    Code: _____

68. Constipation.

    Code: _____

69. Biliary cirrhosis.

    Code: _____

70. Phimosis.

    Code: _____

71. Pyelitis due to tuberculosis.

    Code(s): _____ _____

72. Amenorrhea.

    Code: _____

73. A 24-year-old woman at 28 weeks' gestation has hypothyroidism.

    Code(s): _____ _____

74. A 26-year-old woman at 30 weeks' gestation with quadruplets.

    Code: _____

75. Cellulitis left foot and ankle due to staphylococcus.

    Code(s): _____ _____ _____

76. Systemic lupus erythematosus.

    Code: _____

77. Decubitus ulcer of the sacrum.

    Code: _____

78. Winter itch.

    Code: _____

79. Hidradenitis suppurativa.

    Code: _____

80. Arthritis due to ulcerative colitis.

    Code(s): _____ _____

81. Osteoarthritis of the cervical spine.

    Code: _____

82. Calcaneal spur.

    Code: _____

83. Bunion right big toe.

    Code: _____

84. Acute osteomyelitis left patella due to staphylococcus.

    Code(s): _____ _____

85. Newborn female delivered in the hospital by cesarean delivery with evidence of cleft palate and cleft lip.

    Code(s): _____ _____

86. Chronic osteomyelitis of the hip.

    Code: _____

87. Hepatomegaly.

    Code: _____

88. Epistaxis.

    Code: _____

89. Proteinuria.

    Code: _____

90. Nausea and vomiting.

    Code: _____

91. Polydipsia.

    Code: _____

92. Palpitations due to overdose of monoamine oxidase.

    Code(s): _____ _____ _____

93. Fracture, right clavicle.

    Code: _____

94. Sprain, left ankle.

    Code: _____

95. Abrasion, right elbow.

    Code: _____

96. First- and second-degree burn, forehead.

    Code: _____

97. Concussion.

    Code: _____

98. Foreign body (penny) in stomach.

    Code(s): _____ _____

99. Contusion, left hip.

    Code: _____

100. Traumatic amputation, right foot without complications.

    Code: _____

101. Posterior dislocation of elbow, closed.

    Code: _____

102. Amputation of the left arm just above the elbow.

    Code: _____

103. A patient develops gastrointestinal bleeding while taking Motrin as prescribed for abdominal cramping. (Hint: Two conditions need to be coded. You will need to consult the *Physicians' Desk Reference* to find out what Motrin is called in its generic form.)

    Code(s): _____ _____

104. A patient is admitted with nausea, weakness, sweating, and tachycardia following a gastrectomy. A diagnosis of dumping syndrome is made.

    a. The condition here is dumping syndrome. What is the code for this condition?

    Code: _____

    b. Why is the code 997.4, gastrointestinal complications, not correct

    to assign? _____

105. Acute renal failure develops in a patient following a cardiac catheterization and the patient is admitted for dialysis.

    a. There are two conditions in the case. What are they?

    _____

    b. What are the two codes for these conditions?

    Code(s): _____ _____

106. A patient died from an accidental overdose of heroin. (Hint: Use the Table of Drugs and Chemicals and assign an E code.) What are the codes?

    Code(s): _____ _____

107. A patient is lethargic with severe abdominal cramping and vomiting following an accidental ingestion of 5 tablets of Tylenol with codeine and a bottle of vodka. There are nine codes for this case:

    a. Codeine, poisoning.

    Code(s): _____ _____

    b. Acetaminophen, poisoning.

    Code(s): _____ _____

    c. Alcohol, beverage.

    Code(s): _____ _____

d. Lethargy.

Code: _____

e. Vomiting.

Code: _____

f. Cramp, abdominal, unspecified site.

Code: _____

108. Positive occult blood in stools.

Code: _____

Remember the ♘ symbol means the answer may be one code or more than one code.

109. ASHD of native coronary artery and COPD.

♘ Code(s): _____

110. Candidal endocarditis.

♘ Code(s): _____

111. Pneumonia due to staphylococcus aureus.

♘ Code(s): _____

112. Bacteremia due to pseudomonas.

♘ Code(s): _____

113. Type II cerebral poliomyelitis with dysphonia.

♘ Code(s): _____

114. First-degree sunburn.

♘ Code(s): _____

115. Contusion of the buttock after slipping on the ice.

♘ Code(s): _____

116. MMR immunization.

♘ Code(s): _____

117. Malignant ascites, primary site unknown.

♘ Code(s): _____

118. Stiffness of the knee.

♘ Code(s): _____

119. Dehiscence of the internal wires after sternotomy.

    Code(s): _____

120. Progressive malignant anemia.

    Code(s): _____

121. Alcoholic delirium tremors.

    Code(s): _____

122. Organic personality syndrome.

    Code(s): _____

123. Welder's keratitis (an E code is also required).

    Code(s): _____

124. Transient visual loss.

    Code(s): _____

125. Bilateral otitis media.

    Code(s): _____

126. Idiopathic migraine due to menstruation.

    Code(s): _____

127. Retained foreign body of the lens.

    Code(s): _____

128. Type II diabetic mononeuropathy of the legs.

    Code(s): _____

129. Diarrhea due to paracolon bacillus.

    Code(s): _____

130. Mobitz II atrioventricular block.

    Code(s): _____

131. Suspected carrier of diphtheria.

    Code(s): _____

132. Congenital splenomegaly causing fevers.

    Code(s): _____

133. Dissecting abdominal aortic aneurysm.

   Code(s): _____

134. Cardiac insufficiency 6 months after coronary artery bypass surgery.

   Code(s): _____

135. Raynaud's syndrome with gangrene of right index finger.

   Code(s): _____

136. Ulcerated internal hemorrhoids.

   Code(s): _____

137. Deep vein thrombophlebitis of the femoral vein.

   Code(s): _____

138. Viral pneumonia.

   Code(s): _____

139. Peptic ulcer, bleeding.

   Code(s): _____

140. Impacted wisdom tooth.

   Code(s): _____

141. Colostomy malfunction.

   Code(s): _____

142. Allergic gastritis secondary to aspirin intake, aspirin prescribed for arthritis.

   Code(s): _____

143. Endometriosis of the ovary and round ligament.

   Code(s): _____

144. Chronic prostatitis due to staphylococcus.

   Code(s): _____

145. Stress urinary incontinence, female.

   Code(s): _____

146. Benign prostatic hypertrophy.

   Code(s): _____

147. Pain of the ribs.

   🌀 Code(s): _____

148. Term pregnancy, delivered live born, with preeclampsia and fetal distress.

   🌀 Code(s): _____

149. Impetigo of eyelid.

   🌀 Code(s): _____

150. Systemic lupus erythematosus with lung involvement.

   🌀 Code(s): _____

151. Marble bones.

   🌀 Code(s): _____

152. Arthritis of the hip, status post hip fracture 5 years ago.

   🌀 Code(s): _____

153. Localized osteoarthritis of the wrist.

   🌀 Code(s): _____

154. Patient comes into the ER unconscious.

   🌀 Code(s): _____

155. Adult respiratory distress after falling out of a tree and striking chest on the ground.

   🌀 Code(s): _____

156. Deep cut on the finger embedded with dirt.

   🌀 Code(s): _____

157. Intrinsic obstruction of the eustachian tube.

   🌀 Code(s): _____

158. Obstructive jaundice.

   🌀 Code(s): _____

159. Elevated blood pressure in a patient with hypertension.

   🌀 Code(s): _____

160. Respiratory distress.

   🌀 Code(s): _____

161. Left lower quadrant abdominal tenderness.

    Code(s): _____

162. Pathological fracture of two vertebrae.

    Code(s): _____

163. Splinter of the left palm of the hand.

    Code(s): _____

164. Lung nodule.

    Code(s): _____

165. Second-degree burn of the hand.

    Code(s): _____

166. Accidental overdose of ibuprofen.

    Code(s): _____

167. Second-degree burn of the arm caused by hot water.

    Code(s): _____

168. Status post intracerebral hemorrhage secondary to head injury 1 year ago.

    Code(s): _____

169. Occlusion of renal dialysis graft.

    Code(s): _____

170. Abrasion of leg without infection.

    Code(s): _____

171. Wood splinter in the fingertip.

    Code(s): _____

172. Concussion with 2-hour loss of consciousness.

    Code(s): _____

173. Hemochromatosis.

    Code(s): _____

174. Respiratory arrest of the newborn.

    Code(s): _____

175. Patient admitted to donate bone marrow for brother with aplastic anemia (used by facility coder only).

    Code(s): _____

176. Exposure to rabies.

    Code(s): _____

177. Closure of colostomy (used by facility coder only).

    Code(s): _____

178. Epigastric abdominal pain.

    Code(s): _____

179. Elevated glucose tolerance test.

    Code(s): _____

180. Reprogramming of cardiac pacemaker.

    Code(s): _____

PRINCIPAL DIAGNOSIS

Provide the principal diagnosis and code(s) and any additional diagnoses and code(s) for the following:

181. **HISTORY OF PRESENT ILLNESS:** The patient is a 52-year-old male who was involved in an interpersonal altercation at approximately 1:30 in the morning. He presented to the emergency department with complaints of pain and swelling to the right side of the face. The patient had been struck multiple times with the butt end of a handgun. He denied loss of consciousness. The attack was witnessed, and the witnesses also claimed there was no loss of consciousness. He presented with pain and swelling on the right side of his face in the temporal region and in the right eye region. He had a small abrasion on the top of his head and on the right forehead. No lacerations were noted. He had no diplopia. The past medical history and past surgical history were noncontributory. The patient was taking no medications and had no allergies.

HOSPITAL COURSE: Admission x-rays and CT scan revealed a nondisplaced right zygoma fracture and an orbital floor fracture with slight limitation on physical examination of his upward gaze.

He was taken to the operating room for exploration and placement of a Silastic implant to the right orbital floor fracture, which was accomplished without difficulty and without complication. The patient tolerated the procedure well. Postoperative course was uncomplicated. He received IV antibiotics throughout his stay in the hospital.

FINAL DIAGNOSIS: Right orbital fracture; right zygoma fracture; abrasion of head.

PRINCIPAL DIAGNOSIS and CODE(S): _____

OTHER DIAGNOSES and CODE(S): _____

PROCEDURE CODE(S): _____

182. **HISTORY OF PRESENT ILLNESS:** The patient is a 69-year-old, right-handed male who presents with a 4-day history of severe right-sided headache, visual blurring, and diplopia. The patient was seen in the ENT clinic for discharge from his right ear of 2 days' duration, diagnosed to be otitis externa on the day of admission. The patient was subsequently transferred from the clinic to the emergency department. The patient denied a history of seizure, motor or sensory deficit, nausea or vomiting, trauma, or speech difficulties. Past medical history of sinusitis for many years. Current medications are none. Allergies, none.

PHYSICAL EXAMINATION:
HEENT: Right pupil 3 mm, nonreactive. Left pupil 2 mm, reactive. Disconjugate gaze present. Right ptosis. Oropharynx clear without lesions. The neck is supple without lymphadenopathy or thyromegaly. Heart: regular rate and rhythm without murmurs or gallops. Lungs clear to percussion and auscultation. The neurological examination: awake, alert, oriented times three, follows three simple commands. Cranial nerves, partial right third nerve palsy with ptosis, 3-mm

nonreactive right pupil, right medial gaze with disconjugate extraocular eye movement. Motor is 5/5 throughout without drift. Finger test is within normal limits. The sensory is intact to fine touch and proprioception: cerebral examination within normal limits.

HOSPITAL COURSE: Patient was admitted with suspicion of intracranial aneurysm. On the following day, the patient underwent a three-vessel cerebral angiogram that demonstrated a posterior communicating artery aneurysm and questionable anterior communicating artery aneurysm. The patient underwent a right craniotomy for clipping of right posterior communicating artery aneurysm and anterior communicating artery aneurysm. Postoperatively, the patient was observed in the surgical intensive care unit until his mental status was stabilized. The palsy and ptosis noted preoperatively resolved during the postsurgical course. The patient has been ambulating without assistance and tolerating food well. The patient was also seen by the ENT service during the hospitalization for his otitis externa and their recommendations were followed.

FINAL DIAGNOSES: Right posterior communicating artery aneurysm; anterior communicating artery aneurysm; right otitis externa.

PRINCIPAL DIAGNOSIS and CODE(S): _____

OTHER DIAGNOSES and CODE(S): _____

PROCEDURE CODE(S): _____

SEQUENCING EXERCISES

Cases of Principal Diagnosis and Other Diagnoses

In the following cases, identify the principal diagnosis and other diagnoses using the official coding guidelines. This is not a coding exercise; it is a sequencing exercise.

183. Mr. Jones presents to the emergency department with complaints of leg pain, inflammation and swelling of the ankle and calf, and a fever. The day before he had been seen in the physician's office for treatment of cellulitis and was given antibiotics. Mr. Jones was admitted to the hospital for IV antibiotics.

    Principal Diagnosis: _____

    Other Diagnoses: _____

184. Mrs. Beatty was seen in her physician's office with a complaint of shortness of breath and chest pain. Dr. Adams admitted her with a diagnosis of congestive heart failure.

    Principal Diagnosis: _____

    Other Diagnoses: _____

185. Mr. Janes was admitted for colon resection for colon cancer and also had chemotherapy following surgery. Mr. Janes complained of joint pain while in the hospital, and an MRI showed metastases to bone.

    Principal Diagnosis: _____

    Other Diagnoses: _____

186. Mrs. Anderson had a hysterectomy and bilateral oophorectomy for ovarian cancer 1 week ago. It is planned that the patient will undergo chemotherapy. The patient is now admitted with internal hemorrhaging from surgery site.

    Principal Diagnosis: _____

    Other Diagnoses: _____

187. Miss Nelson is admitted for a D&C for menorrhagia. During her preoperative physical examination, the physician notices she has a fever and her lungs are congested. He cancels surgery because the patient shows symptoms of acute bronchitis.

    Principal Diagnosis: _____

    Other Diagnoses: _____

188. Jackie Jones was cooking at home and spilled a pot of boiling water on her arms, legs, and stomach. She presented to the emergency department with second-degree burns of the thighs and third-degree

burns of the arms and stomach. She was admitted and taken directly to surgery.

Principal Diagnosis: _____

Other Diagnoses: _____

189. Mr. Anderson regularly sees a physician and is on medication for management of his chronic bronchitis. Last night he was complaining of coughing and difficulty breathing. He was admitted with a diagnosis of chronic bronchitis with acute exacerbation.

Principal Diagnosis: _____

Other Diagnoses: _____

190. Mrs. Smith is at 32 weeks' gestation and complaining of stomach cramps and diarrhea × 36 hours. She is admitted for rehydration with IV fluids and is diagnosed with dehydration and gastroenteritis. Pregnancy is felt to be incidental.

Principal Diagnosis: _____

Other Diagnoses: _____

REPORTS

Toward the end of this textbook, you will find a section titled Reports, which contains original reports. Read the reports indicated below and supply the appropriate ICD-9-CM codes (both diagnoses and Volume 3 procedure codes) on the following lines:

191. Report 6 🐚   Code(s): _____

192. Report 7 🐚   Code(s): _____

193. Report 8 🐚   Code(s): _____

194. Report 9 🐚   Code(s): _____

195. Report 10 🐚   Code(s): _____

196. Report 11 🐚   Code(s): _____

197. Report 12 🐚   Code(s): _____

198. Report 13 🐚   Code(s): _____

199. Report 14 🐚   Code(s): _____

200. Report 15 🐚   Code(s): _____

201. Report 19 🐚   Code(s): _____

202. Report 20 🐚   Code(s): _____

203. Report 28 🐚   Code(s): _____

204. Report 31 🐚   Code(s): _____

205. Report 32 🐚   Code(s): _____

206. Report 33 🐚   Code(s): _____

207. Report 34 🐚   Code(s): _____

208. Report 35 🐚   Code(s): _____

209. Report 36 🐚   Code(s): _____

210. Report 38 🐚   Code(s): _____

211. Report 39 🐚   Code(s): _____

212. Report 41 🐚   Code(s): _____

213. Report 42 🐚   Code(s): _____

214. Report 43 🐚   Code(s): _____

215. Report 44 🐚   Code(s): _____

CHAPTER 16

Third-Party Reimbursement Issues

THEORY

Without the use of reference material, answer the following:

1. What two groups of persons were added to those eligible for Medicare benefits after the initial establishment of the Medicare program?

   a. _____

   b. _____

2. To what government organization did the Secretary of the Department of Health and Human Services delegate the responsibility for administering the Medicare program?

   _____

3. What government organization handles the funds for the Medicare program?

   _____

4. There are three items that Medicare beneficiaries are responsible for paying before Medicare will begin to pay for services. What are these three items?

   _____, _____, and _____

5. Each of the DRGs is defined by a set of six patient attributes, which include:

_____, _____, _____,

_____, _____, _____

6. How many MDCs are there? _____

7. What two things are defined as a condition that increased the patient's length of stay in the hospital by at least 1 day in at least 75% of the patients?

_____ and _____

8. What age is sometimes used in the DRG definition of the patients?

_____

9. What are three DRGs that are used to indicate the patient had a surgery unrelated to the principal diagnosis?

_____, _____, and _____

10. What are MDC flowcharts also called? _____

11. Medicare publishes the Medicare fee schedule and usually pays what percentage of the amounts indicated for services? _____

12. The three components of work, overhead, and malpractice are part of an RVU. What do the initials RVU stand for? _____

_____

13. According to the Physician Payment Reform, providers must file claims for their Medicare patients within what time period?

_____

14. What is the term that is used in the APC system to refer to the inclusion of certain ancillary services into the payment for the visit?

_____

15. How many days' notice did CMS give before implementation of APCs?

_____

16. The APC system consists of how many groups of services?

_____

17. The APC coinsurance amount for beneficiaries is based on what percent of the national median charge? _____

18. Hospitals submit inpatient charges to Medicare using what codes?

    _____

19. What edition of the *Federal Register* would the hospitals be especially interested in?

    _____

20. What editions of the *Federal Register* would the outpatient facilities be interested in?

    _____ _____ and _____

21. Where and when did the design and development of the DRGs begin?

    _____

22. What was the first state to use the DRG system on a wide scale?

    _____

23. Some hospitals justified their higher costs of patient care by stating that they treated what type of patients? _____

24. The concept of case mix complexity has been used to refer to a set of five patient attributes. Name three of the five.

    _____

    _____

    _____

25. What does MDC stand for? _____

    _____ _____

26. Explain what is considered a substantial complication or comorbidity within the DRG system.

    _____

    _____

    _____

27. Under what act were the PROs made possible? _____

28. Under what act was a major change in Medicare in 1989 made possible?

    _____

29. Can a physician charge a patient to complete a Medicare form?

    _____

APPENDIX A

Reports

1. EMERGENCY DEPARTMENT REPORT

The patient is a 32-year-old G-5, P-4, female at 36 weeks and 4 days by last menstrual period, who comes in to the emergency room complaining of a 4-day history of urinary frequency and urgency with cloudy urine. She is also complaining of some low back pain × 5 days. She denies burning, itching, pain with urination. She denies fever and chills. She has also had some nausea and vomiting over the same period. She last vomited yesterday. She vomited twice, she states, and, this past Friday, 4 days ago, twice. She has not vomited today. She has had good fluid intake. She has had a slightly decreased appetite, she states. The patient states that she has had some UTIs this pregnancy × 2. Otherwise, she has had an uncomplicated pregnancy.

The patient denies a history of hypertension, diabetes, and preeclampsia. She states she has had some irregular contractions, no real contractions today. She denies vaginal bleeding. She denies gush of fluid. She denies abdominal pain. She has had good fetal movement. She has not had headaches, visual changes, or abdominal pain.

PHYSICAL EXAMINATION: Blood pressure 119/66, temperature 36.5, pulse 86, respiratory rate 18. HEENT: Within normal limits. CHEST: Clear to auscultation bilaterally. HEART: Regular rate and rhythm without murmur, rub, or gallop. ABDOMEN: Gravida, nontender. Vertex. EXTREMITIES: The patient has 1+ pitting edema bilaterally to the knee. On cervical examination, the patient was 1-2 cm, long, −1 station. Fetal heart tones are 130's with accels. No obvious contractions on the monitor. No flank tenderness to palpation.

LABORATORY DATA: Urinalysis is done and revealed yellow, turbid urine, specific gravity of 1.022, 100 protein, positive nitrite, moderate hemoglobin, large amount of leukocytes, 5-10 red cells, 3+ bacteria, too numerous to count white cells.

ASSESSMENT: This is a 32-year-old, G-5, P-4 at 36 and 4/5 weeks, with a urinary tract infection. The patient was given a prescription for Macrobid 100 mg p.o. b.i.d. × 7 days. She is instructed to follow up with her OB doctor in 2 days for recheck of her urine and her symptomatology. She was given labor precautions. She was advised that, if she develops fevers, back pain, worsening symptomatology, she should come in immediately for evaluation.

2. DISCHARGE SUMMARY

DIAGNOSES include:

1. Chronic pelvic pain secondary to pelvic metastatic clear cell carcinoma of unknown primary location.
2. Vena cava syndrome post placement of Hickman catheter.
3. Anemia of chronic disease.
4. Hypertension.

HOSPITAL COURSE: The patient is a 78-year-old female whom we have been following in our clinic for hypertension and also chronic pudendal nerve pain. She had been recently diagnosed with pelvic metastatic clear cell carcinoma which her primary location is unknown at this time. She will be discussing this further after the pathology reports are read. During her hospital stay a Hickman catheter was placed in order to have IV access for pain medication or future cancer therapy. She was also admitted for chronic pain. She did develop swelling of her arms and neck. She was brought to interventional radiology and she did have venography and the Hickman catheter was removed. Her swelling to her arms and neck have decreased greatly. She denies any shortness of breath. No choking sensation as previously noted. Her pain has been managed well with fentanyl patch at 175 mcg. She has also been on IV heparin therapy for anticoagulation following the vena cava syndrome. Today, the patient has been having complaints of nausea. She did get some dexamethasone IV for her nausea which did improve later this morning. Her blood pressure has been under good control. Her labs today include a WBC of 5.18, hemoglobin 7.8, hematocrit 23.7, protime 14.4, INR 1.5, PTT is 39.6, BUN 6, sodium 139, potassium 4.2, C02 27.2.

DISCHARGE PLANS:

1. IV heparin is discontinued. She will be switched over to Lovenox 1 mg/kg subcutaneously daily. The patient will have Home Health to help her setup these injections.
2. She will continue with the fentanyl patch 175 mcg for the pain.
3. She will receive 40,000 units subcutaneously of Procrit at the Cancer Center one time per week. We will follow up in 3 days with a CBC and a basic metabolic panel.
4. Follow-up appointment at the Kidney and Hypertension Center on November 2 at 10:30 in the morning. Will also check CBC and a basic metabolic panel, PTT, PT and INR before that appointment.
5. Hold potassium supplements for now.
6. She may use Phenergan p.o. 12.5 mg 1-2 tablets p.o. p.r.n. every 6 hours for nausea.
7. She does have a follow-up appointment setup with Dr. Noyes on Friday, 10/29/04 to discuss her pathology results and decide what further treatment is to be done. He will also be discussing plans with Dr. Sticca.

The above plan was discussed with the patient and her husband. They seem to be in agreement. They were encouraged to call our office with any questions or concerns.

DISCHARGE MEDICATIONS:

1. Will continue home medications.
2. Phenergan 12.5 1-2 tabs p.o. p.r.n. every 6 hours for nausea.
3. Lovenox 1 mg/kg subcutaneously every 24 hours.
4. Fentanyl patch 175 mcg to be changed every 3 days.
5. Epogen 40,000 units subcutaneously weekly at the Cancer Center.

Total time spent with the patient today is 60 minutes.

3. CLINIC CHART NOTE

HISTORY: This 16-year-old female is seen today after falling off a curb and twisting her right ankle. She is normally a patient of Dr. Anderson, who is out of town this week. (Both physicians are of the same specialty and in the same clinic.) She states that she has pain surrounding the entire foot and ankle. Seems unable or unwilling to bear weight. (Problem-focused history)

PHYSICAL EXAMINATION: Ankle and foot examined. Foot is warm to touch. Some swelling and bruising noted around the lateral aspect of the ankle. X-ray is negative for fracture. (Problem-focused examination)

IMPRESSION: Sprained right ankle. (MDM complexity straightforward)

PLAN: Elevation; ice to affected area. Weight bearing only as tolerated. Return for follow-up prn.

4. ADMIT INPATIENT

This is a 19-year-old with a living-related donor kidney transplant as of last month and admitted to hospital for possible sepsis.

HISTORY: This patient has type 1 diabetes and had been on dialysis for a number of years before transplantation. She received her mother's kidney on the 14th of last month from the Medical Center Transplant Program in Dallas. She was there this Tuesday for a transplant visit and apparently did not feel well, but they were not certain whether this was a problem or not; but they did go ahead and do blood cultures and called the public health nurse, who was visiting the patient today, and said that one of the cultures was positive for group B strep. The home health nurse called me and stated that the patient has really gone downhill the past few days and was quite fatigued with generalized malaise. Denied cough, fever, or shaking chills but looked poor overall, and the nurse was quite concerned. We recommended she be brought here for evaluation and treatment as an emergency. After arrival here, she was in no acute distress. Initially, she had bibasilar crackles on deep breathing; however, most of these cleared. I cannot hear any significant pulmonary abnormality on auscultation or percussion. Her heart is normal regular rhythm. No significant murmurs, rubs, S3, or S4. Her abdomen is negative. Her left lower-quadrant kidney is nontender. She has no edema and no lateralizing neural sounds. She is a little lethargic. She does not feel warm. Apparently she is afebrile. Her blood pressure is normal, and she is not tachycardic, but she simply does not look well. Past history, social history, and system review are per our recent old chart and noncontributory at present.

MEDICATIONS: See med sheet.

CLINCAL IMPRESSION: One positive group B strep blood culture, significance, and/or etiology to be determined. My impression at this time is probably a significant finding and suspect that this will become a progressive syndrome if not treated.

ADDITIONAL DIAGNOSES:

1. Living-related donor kidney transplant
2. Diabetes mellitus type 1
3. Hypertension

PLAN: Repeat culture. Culture urine. Do chest x-ray stat and repeat lab. Will empirically treat pending results at this time.

5. NEPHROLOGY HOSPITAL PROGRESS NOTE

This patient continues to be stable with no new problems. Her cultures remain negative, and she remains afebrile. Her clearance is pending, but she certainly has settled down nicely. The main problem we are having is with her diabetic management. It simply is not working with the former twice a day of 70/30 insulin plus a nighttime Lantus. I think we should go one way or the other, and we will go to Humalog before each meal, starting with an estimated dose of 15 per meal and 40 of Lantus in the evening, and we will titrate from there. We will get Accu-Cheks before each meal to reflect the previous meal's dose of Humalog and adjust it accordingly. Other than that, tomorrow we will review her case with infectious disease with regard to the duration of her antibiotic therapy. Thus far, our cultures have remained negative; however, the positive group B strep is not the type of typical contaminant you get in a blood culture, and we must take it at face value.

Time spent reevaluating the patient, reviewing the chart, and rearranging diabetic management was 25 minutes.

6. OPERATIVE REPORT

PREOPERATIVE DIAGNOSIS: Scar right parietal region.

POSTOPERATIVE DIAGNOSIS: Same.

SURGICAL FINDINGS: 3×1 cm elevated scar right parietal region of scalp.

SURGICAL PROCEDURE: Excision scar of scalp.

SURGEON:

ANESTHESIA: General endotracheal anesthesia, plus 2 cc of 1% Xylocaine and 1:100,000 epinephrine.

PROCEDURE: The scalp was prepped with Betadine scrub and solution, draped in the routine sterile fashion. The lesion was anesthetized with 2 cc of 1% Xylocaine with 1:100,000 epinephrine, mostly for the epinephrine effect. After a wait of 4 minutes the lesion was excised, bleeding was electrocoagulated, the wound was closed with vertical mattress sutures of 3-0 Prolene. Surgicel and antibiotic ointment were applied. The patient tolerated the procedure well and left the operating room in good condition.

PATHOLOGY REPORT LATER INDICATED: See Report 64.

7. OPERATIVE REPORT

PREOPERATIVE DIAGNOSIS: Lipoma left posterior axillary fold.

POSTOPERATIVE DIAGNOSIS: Same.

SURGICAL FINDINGS: 6 cm diameter lipoma attached to latissimus dorsi muscle.

PROCEDURE PERFORMED: Excision of lipoma left posterior axillary fold.

ANESTHESIA: General endotracheal anesthesia with 5 cc 1% Xylocaine with 1:100,000 epinephrine injected along the incision line.

COMPLICATIONS: None.

SPONGE AND NEEDLE COUNT: Correct.

DRAINS: One #10 Jackson Pratt.

DESCRIPTION OF PROCEDURE: The patient's posterior arm was prepped with Betadine scrub and solution and draped in the routine sterile fashion. About 5 cc of 1% Xylocaine with 1:100,000 epinephrine were injected along the incision line. Dissection was carried down to the site of the lipomatous mass which was dissected free of the skin and dissected free of the muscle using sharp dissection with very little bleeding. Bleeding was electrocoagulated. Because of the size of the pocket, we inserted a drain and brought it out through a separate stab wound incision using a #10 Jackson Pratt drain. The wound was then closed, effectively closing the dead space with interrupted 2-0 Monocryl, subcuticular 3-0 Monocryl and a few twists of 4-0 Prolene. Dressing consisted of Kerlix fluffs, Elastoplast, a clavicle strap and a sling. The patient tolerated the procedure well and left the area in good condition.

PATHOLOGY REPORT LATER INDICATED: See Report 60.

8. OPERATIVE REPORT

PREOPERATIVE DIAGNOSIS: Pyelogenic granuloma, sinus tract, buttock.

POSTOPERATIVE DIAGNOSIS: Multiple sinus tracts, one extending inferiorly about 7 × 3 cm in diameter, one extending to the right approximately 4 × 3 cm, and one extending to the left for about 3 cm.

SURGICAL FINDINGS: As above, plus (benign) granulation tissue present in a capsule of multiple sinus tracts. Sinus tracts measured a total of about 15 × 8 cm in their total dimensions.

SURGICAL PROCEDURE: Partial unroofing of sinus tracts.

ANESTHESIA: General endotracheal.

DESCRIPTION OF PROCEDURE: The patient intubated and turned in the prone position. A probe was inserted in the sinus cavity, and dissection was carried down to this. I encountered a piece of chronically infected granulation tissue coming out of a hole, in which I stuck the probe, but this continued for a distance longer than the probe and accordingly, I put my finger in this and this extended down the length of my index finger (i.e., about 7–8 cm by about 3 cm in width). I left this intact, because this would necessitate extensive dissection and we have no blood on this patient at this time. We then unroofed two other sinus cavities, and packed this opened with 2-inch vaginal packing and applied a dressing and Kerlix plus an

Elastoplast. Estimated blood loss: 25 cc. The patient seemed to tolerate the procedure well and left the operating room in good condition.

9. OPERATIVE REPORT

PREOPERATIVE DIAGNOSIS: Mass, right breast.

POSTOPERATIVE DIAGNOSIS: Mass, right breast.

OPERATIVE PROCEDURE: Right breast mass excision.

PROCEDURE: With the patient under general anesthesia, the breast and chest were prepped and draped in a sterile manner. An elliptical incision was made about the palpated mass, including the area of the nipple. This was excised all the way down to the fascia of the breast and then submitted for frozen section. Frozen section revealed a carcinoma of the breast with what appeared to be a good margin all the way around it. We then maintained hemostasis with electrocautery and proceeded to close the breast tissue using 2-0 and 3-0 chromic. The skin was closed using 4-0 Vicryl in a subcuticular manner. Steri-Strips were applied. The patient tolerated the procedure well and was discharged from the operating room in stable condition.

PATHOLOGY REPORT LATER INDICATED: Primary, malignant neoplasm.

10. OPERATIVE REPORT

PREOPERATIVE DIAGNOSIS: Neck injury, motor vehicle accident.

POSTOPERATIVE DIAGNOSIS: Same as preoperative.

PROCEDURE PERFORMED: Placement of halo crown and vest.

ANESTHESIA: Local.

SURGICAL INDICATIONS: This 56-year-old patient was in a motor vehicle accident and appears to have sustained a spinal cord injury with ligamentous instability at C4-5. He could not be placed in a neck collar because he has a short thick neck and also because he had a tracheostomy tube. The patient would not be stabilized with traction as he has a distraction injury. It was indicated to place him in a halo vest and crown to immobilize his neck.

PROCEDURE: The hair was shaved behind both ears. There was a sterile prep done along the forehead region and the region behind both ears. The halo crown was then positioned and stabilized with the three positioners anteriorly and two laterally. I then injected Xylocaine behind both ears and along the supraorbital ridge laterally. I then placed the four pins and torqued them to 8 pounds per sq inch. The hexagonal lock nuts were then tightened. The patient tolerated this well without any apparent complications. The halo vest was then connected to the crown. The crown was placed. A large vest was used but this was still too small for the patient, and on the right side the vest had to be tied with string until some permanent straps could be fashioned by orthotics. During the placement of the vest, I maintained the neck in neutral position and at no time was there any rotation or flexion or extension of the neck.

11. OPERATIVE REPORT

PREOPERATIVE DIAGNOSIS: Bulky free flap, right heel.

POSTOPERATIVE DIAGNOSIS: Same.

SURGICAL FINDINGS: 10.5 × 8.5 cm area of redundant fat of flap of right heel.

PROCEDURE PERFORMED: Defatting of flap of right heel with excision of redundant skin (benign).

ANESTHESIA: General endotracheal anesthesia

POSITION: Prone

ESTIMATED BLOOD LOSS: Negligible

DESCRIPTION OF PROCEDURE: The patient was intubated and turned into prone position. The right foot and lower leg were prepped with Betadine scrub and solution and was draped in the routine sterile fashion. The medial aspect of the flap was elevated excising the old scar in the process, and the flap was elevated to about 60% of its extent to include all of the redundant fat that was within the flap. We removed about 1.5 cm thickness of flap from the bottom of the flap and left a layer of padding of about a cm on the bed. Hemostasis was secured, and then we closed the wound with a combination of plain 3-0 Prolene and horizontal mattress sutures and some horizontal half mattress sutures of 3-0 Prolene. We dressed the wound temporarily with Kerlix and Kling and Dr. Miller will then proceed with his portion of the procedure.

12. OPERATIVE REPORT

PREOPERATIVE DIAGNOSIS: Ischial ulcer with massive ischioperineal and buttock sinus.

POSTOPERATIVE DIAGNOSIS: Same.

FINDINGS: There was a 2 cm open surgical ulcer extending down and connecting with an 8 × 30 cm diameter granulation-lined sinus cavity.

SURGICAL PROCEDURE: Excision of left ischial ulcer with total excision of 8 × 30 cm sinus of the buttock, perineal and ischial areas.

ANESTHESIA: General endotracheal.

ESTIMATED BLOOD LOSS: 400 mL.

FLUIDS: 2 liters Ringer's lactate.

DRAINS: None.

COMPLICATION: None.

SPONGE AND NEEDLE COUNTS: Correct

DESCRIPTION: The patient was intubated and turned in the right lateral decubitus position. I injected about 10 mL of 1% Xylocaine with 1:100,000 epinephrine around the surface ulcer, and made incisions down to the granulation tissue, keeping this intact. I opened the skin over the extent of the sinus tracts proximally and distally, trying to keep this in line with a potential Y-V advancement flap, and with some difficulty and remarkable bleeding around what appeared to be the sacrum, I was able to remove virtually intact the entire ulcer, covered with chronically infected granulation tissue. This granulation tissue was poor quality and had an unhealthy appearance. A piece of this was dropped in a culture tube as was a piece of what appeared to be the sacrum, which was quite sclerotic and consistent with an osteomyelitis of the sacrum. Following this extensive removal of the ulcer, I cauterized all of the bleeding and did a stick-tie on one of the bleeders with 2-0 Vicryl. I then sprayed the base with topical thrombin, packed the wound open with 2″ vaginal packing soaked in 5/10th percent metronidazole, and then put several #2 Prolene sutures to keep the packing in place and to help seal off the wound from the fecal contamination. I put a Vi-Drape over this and then dressed it with Kerlix fluffs, ABD pads and Elastoplast. The patient tolerated the procedure well and left the area in good condition.

PATHOLOGY REPORT LATER INDICATED: See Report 62.

13. OPERATIVE REPORT

PROCEDURE: Steroid injection.

INDICATIONS: Left shoulder subacromial bursitis.

PROCEDURE: This procedure was done in the procedure area in the hospital. After obtaining consent, area of the left shoulder was prepped in the usual fashion with Betadine. 6 cc of 1% lidocaine with 1 cc of Kenalog was injected in the left subacromial bursa without difficulty. The patient tolerated the procedure well without immediate complications. There was moderate relief of pain afterward. The patient was advised to call me if she gets any signs of infection, such as fever, chills, erythema, or swelling. She will call me in 3 days and tell me how she is doing.

14. OPERATIVE REPORT

PREOPERATIVE DIAGNOSIS: Neurologic, neuromuscular dysfunction.

POSTOPERATIVE DIAGNOSIS: Same.

PRELIMINARY NOTE: This patient was brought down to the operating room on the ventilator and we used the operating room because of this.

OPERATIVE NOTE: With the patient in the supine position we prepped and draped the left deltoid region. After infiltration with 0.5% Marcaine with epinephrine, a vertical incision was made over the palpated muscular belly. Sharp dissection was carried down to the muscle belly and then we freed up a segment of muscle. We did infiltrate the ends of the muscle away from where we were taking our biopsy with the Marcaine. A segment of muscle was then isolated between clamps and then we excised the segment of muscle and submitted it immediately to the histology department for proper processing. The ends of the muscle were ligated using 2-0 chromic and then the muscular fascia was brought together using 2-0 chromic. Subcutaneous tissue was closed using 2-0 chromic and then the skin was closed using 4-0 nylon in running mattress fashion. A sterile dressing was applied. The patient tolerated the procedure well and was discharged from the operating room in stable condition. At the end of the procedure all sponges and instruments were accounted for.

PATHOLOGY REPORT LATER INDICATED: See Report 59.

15. OPERATIVE REPORT

PREOPERATIVE DIAGNOSIS: Left distal radius fracture.

POSTOPERATIVE DIAGNOSIS: Same.

PROCEDURE PERFORMED: Closed reduction and pinning of left distal radius fracture.

COMPLICATIONS: None.

INDICATIONS: This is a 31-year-old female who fell yesterday down a flight of stairs, fracturing her left wrist. She has been stabilized in the intensive care unit throughout the day today. Her injuries include a comminuted intraarticular left distal radius fracture, displaced.

The patient's x-rays are consistent with a displaced comminuted intraarticular distal radius fracture. This is an unstable fracture, and requires reduction and probable pinning versus open reduction and internal fixation.

Prior to the procedure, I spoke with the patient regarding her left wrist. We discussed management options in detail and I recommended proceeding with a closed reduction versus pinning versus ORIF of her left distal radius. The procedure, alternatives, risks, benefits, and expected rehab course were discussed in detail. She understood the implications of surgery and wished to proceed.

PROCEDURE: The patient was brought to the operating room and placed supine on the operating room table. She underwent general anesthesia. The left wrist was initially examined under fluoroscopic guidance. There was comminution and intraarticular involvement. There was dorsal tilt of 30 degrees, shortening, and angulation. We performed a closed reduction with longitudinal traction, manipulation at the fracture, and volar flexion. We obtained a near anatomic reduction with maintenance of radial length and inclination. Additionally, there was neutral tilt. However, with release of traction, there was some instability to the fracture with some residual collapse. Subsequently, the left upper extremity was prepped and draped in standard surgical fashion. Under fluoroscopic guidance, a closed reduction was again obtained. Two separate 0.062 K-wires were placed through the radial styloid, across the main fracture, and into the more proximal shaft. Both of these screws had good fixation in the bone.

Final fluoroscopic views were obtained confirming a near anatomic reduction. The pins were then cut off 1 cm proud to the skin. The pin sites were dressed with Xeroform gauze and adequately padded. The left upper extremity was then placed into a well-padded and molded long arm cast with the wrist in neutral, forearm neutral, and elbow 90 degrees.

The patient was awakened from anesthesia and tolerated the procedure well. She was transferred back to the recovery room in stable condition. There were no intraoperative complications for the wrist portion of the procedure.

16. OPERATIVE REPORT

PREOPERATIVE DIAGNOSIS: Degenerative joint disease, medial compartment plus meniscal tear.

POSTOPERATIVE DIAGNOSIS: Posterior horn tear, medial meniscus; diffuse grade 3–4 chondromalacia, medial femoral condyle 0–90 degrees; and grade 4 chondromalacia, superior half of the patella.

PROCEDURE PERFORMED: Arthroscopy and partial arthroscopic meniscectomy, right knee.

OPERATIVE PROCEDURE: After suitable general anesthesia had been achieved, the patient's right knee was prepped and draped in the usual manner. Before prepping, a thigh tourniquet was applied; after draping, it was inflated to 300 mm Hg. No inflow cannula was used. Arthroscope was inserted through an anteromedial portal. The lateral compartment was examined. Everything looked good. Examination of the notch revealed some inflated synovial tissue, which was cauterized with a radiofrequency probe. Examination of the medial compartment revealed a horizontal cleavage tear and flap tear of the posterior horn of the medial meniscus. Using a combination of punch and shaver, the unstable meniscus was excised and contoured. The tibial surfaces revealed a small area of water by the anterior horn of the meniscus. Femoral surfaces showed diffuse wear of grade 3 with occasional areas of grade 4 chondromalacia from 0–90 degrees. Examination of the patellofemoral joint revealed very good looking articular surfaces on the inferior half of the patella in the trochlea. However, there was essentially bare bone on the superior half of the articular surface.

The knee joint was then thoroughly irrigated, and the arthroscope removed. Stab wounds were closed with 3-0 nylon. A dressing was then applied. Tourniquet was released, after which good circulation was noted to return to the foot. The patient tolerated the procedure well and returned to the recovery room in stable condition.

PATHOLOGY REPORT LATER INDICATED: Benign meniscus tissue and bone chips.

17. OPERATIVE REPORT

PREOPERATIVE DIAGNOSIS: Intertrochanteric/subtrochanteric fracture, right hip.

POSTOPERATIVE DIAGNOSIS: Intertrochanteric/subtrochanteric fracture, right hip.

PROCEDURE PERFORMED: Open reduction internal fixation of intertrochanteric/subtrochanteric fracture, right hip.

ANESTHESIA: Spinal.

FINDINGS: The patient had a displaced comminuted intertrochanteric/subtrochanteric fracture of her right hip. We were able to align this fairly well and hold this in place with a dynamic hip screw device.

PROCEDURE: While under spinal anesthetic, the patient was placed in the supine position on the fracture table, where gentle traction was applied to the right leg and the left leg was abducted. We visualized the fracture using the C-arm image intensifier. We were satisfied with the position and then prepped the patient's right hip with Betadine and draped it in a sterile fashion. She was given 1 g of Kefzol intravenously preoperatively.

We then created a longitudinal incision over the lateral aspect of the right hip and carried the dissection down through the subcutaneous tissue. The fascia was incised longitudinally, and we reflected the vastus lateralis anteriorly, exposing the lateral aspect of the femoral shaft. We were able to palpate the fracture and found that it was significantly displaced. We attempted to reduce this. We then drilled a 9/64-inch hole in the lateral aspect of the femoral shaft through which we advanced a guide pin into the femoral head at an angle of 135 degrees to the femoral shaft. We then passed a reamer over this and reamed to a depth of 110 mm and inserted a 100-mg lag screw into the femoral head. We attempted to position this lag screw in the center of the femoral head as best as possible as seen in both the AP and lateral views.

We then attached a 135-degree four-hole side plate and secured this plate to the femoral shaft using four cortical screws. We then released the traction of the leg and inserted a compressing screw into the end of the lag screw. The resultant fixation appeared to be quite satisfactory. We again used the C-arm image intensifier to evaluate the fracture and found it be very acceptable.

We then thoroughly irrigated the area with saline and placed a Hemovac drain deep to the fascia. We then closed the fascia using 0 Vicryl and the subcutaneous tissue with 2-0 Vicryl. The skin was closed using skin staples. A sterile Xeroform dressing was applied, and the patient was then taken from the operating room in good condition breathing spontaneously. The final sponge and needle counts were correct. She will be continued on IV Kefzol for at least 24 hours.

18. OPERATIVE REPORT

PREOPERATIVE DIAGNOSIS: Comminuted fracture, right olecranon.

POSTOPERATIVE DIAGNOSIS: Comminuted fracture, right olecranon.

PROCEDURE PERFORMED: Open reduction internal fixation, right olecranon fracture.

ANESTHESIA: General.

FINDINGS: The patient had a markedly comminuted displaced fracture of his right olecranon. He had involved a significant portion of the articular surface. We were able to reassemble the major fragments; however, we did have to debride some of the articular cartilage from the joint, which resulted in a defect in the articular cartilage of some significance.

PROCEDURE: While under a general anesthetic, the patient was placed in supine position on the operating room table, where his right arm was prepped with Betadine and draped in a sterile fashion. We used an Esmarch bandage to exsanguinate the arm, and a tourniquet on the limb was inflated to 250 mm Hg. The total tourniquet time ended up being 43 minutes.

We created a longitudinal incision over the posterior aspect of the elbow, skirting to the radial side of the olecranon. We carried the dissection down through the subcutaneous tissue and easily identified the fracture site as the periosteum was torn over this area. We used suction to irrigate the hematoma. Several pieces of articular cartilage lay in the joint, which we debrided, and there was some other cancellous bone, which we debrided as well because it was laying loose in the joint. We then thoroughly irrigated the area with saline to look for any remaining loose fragments. We held this in place with a towel clip as we drilled a transverse hole through the ulna, perhaps 2.5 cm distal to the fracture site. We passed an 18-gauge wire through this transverse tunnel through the ulna, and then we passed two smooth Steinmann pins across the fracture site. We started the Steinmann pins from the proximal fragment and drilled across the fracture site into the distal ulnar shaft. After we had completed the second Steinmann pin across the fracture site, we passed the 18-gauge wire in a figure-of-eight fashion across the fracture site and around the Steinmann pins. We then tightened this with a Harris wire tightener. The combination of the Steinmann pins and the figure-of-eight wire seemed to secure the fracture quite nicely. There was no movement of the fracture site with placing the elbow through a range of motion. We left the Steinmann pins long until we had obtained an intraoperative x-ray confirming an acceptable alignment of the fragment. The x-rays did confirm a significant loss of the articular cartilage; however, it was elected to accept this because the fragments appeared to be relatively stable clinically.

We then bent the Steinmann pins at 90 degrees and cut them off and then taped the Steinmann pins so that they were buried into the triceps muscle. We placed the elbow through a range of motion and found that no crepitus was noted. The fracture appeared to be in good condition, and we therefore irrigated the area with saline and closed the subcutaneous tissue using 2-0 Vicryl and the skin with 3-0 nylon. A Xeroform dressing was applied, and a long-arm splint was applied with the elbow flexed about 60 degrees. He was taken from the operating room in good condition and breathing spontaneously. Tourniquet released after 43 minutes of tourniquet time, and we released this just after the x-rays. He was given IV Kefzol preoperatively and will be continued on IV Kefzol for 24 hours postoperatively as well. The final sponge and needle counts were correct.

19. OPERATIVE REPORT

PREOPERATIVE DIAGNOSIS: Left lung abscess.

POSTOPERATIVE DIAGNOSIS: Same.

PROCEDURE PERFORMED: Left upper lobectomy with decortication and drainage.

INDICATIONS: This 52-year-old female with radiographic evidence of a left upper lobe abscess was admitted the evening before surgery with tension pneumothorax treated with double-lumen intubation and a chest tube. She was subsequently dialyzed to improve hemodynamics and oxygenation, and was felt to be as optimal as possible for her left thoracotomy.

FINDINGS AT SURGERY revealed a large abscess in the left upper lobe accounting for approximately 70% of the left upper lobe parenchyma. Fibrinopurulent exudate was noted on the left lower lobe and throughout the parietal pleural surfaces. This was removed piecemeal with gradual improvement in the left lower lobe pulmonary expansion.

PROCEDURE: The patient was brought to the operating room and placed in the supine position, and under general intubation with a double-lumen tube which had been placed the night before the patient was rolled into the right lateral decubitus position with her left side up. A posterolateral thoracotomy was performed. Adhesions were taken down sharply and bluntly and with cautery. Following this, a standard artery first left upper lobectomy was carried out utilizing 0 silk and hemoclips. The left upper pulmonary vein was secured with a single application of the TA-30 vascular stapling machine. The posterior fissure was created with multiple applications of the TIA automatic stapling machine and the bronchus secured with a single application of the TA-30 bronchus stapling machine. Following this, the wound was drained with three 24-French atrium chest tubes and hemostasis obtained with spray Tisseel, Surgicel gauze. The bronchus was sealed with Bio-glue and the wound closed in layers and a sterile compression dressing applied, and the patient returned to the surgical intensive care unit after changing the double-lumen tube to a single-lumen tube. The patient received 3 units of packed cells intraoperatively to maintain hemostasis. Sponge count and needle count correct ×2.

PATHOLOGY REPORT LATER INDICATED: See Report 65.

20. OPERATIVE REPORT

Endocervical and Endometrial Biopsy

The patient is a 60-year-old married white female, whose last menstrual period was at age 55. No postmenopausal bleeding. Pap is current. Mammogram is not given.

CHIEF COMPLAINT: Metastatic clear cell carcinoma.

The patient is status post CT-guided transgluteal biopsy of a presacral mass which returns as metastatic clear cell carcinoma. Biopsy was performed September 17, 200X. The patient's CT of the abdomen shows the uterus to be slightly enlarged for patient's age, but does not mention ascites or ovarian masses.

MEDICATIONS:

1. Citracal.
2. Lanoxin 0.25 mg.
3. Metoprolol 50 mg b.i.d.
4. Multivitamin.
5. Ocuvite.
6. Xanax.

MEDICAL PROBLEMS:

1. Chronic pelvic pain syndrome.
2. Sacroiliac lipoma.
3. Pudendal neuralgia.
4. Hiatal hernia.

FAMILY HISTORY: Negative.

REVIEW OF SYSTEMS: Positive for glasses, high blood pressure, anxiety, depression.

PROCEDURE: Endocervical and endometrial biopsy.

The patient received antibiotic prophylaxis and then the procedure was performed by visualizing the cervix. The cervix was prepped with Betadine and cytobrush was then used to obtain cervical curetting. The endocervical os was unable to be demonstrated by the Pipelle curette or the uterine sound. The cytobrush was then used to locate the central endometrial canal and the Pipelle curette was then used to obtain endometrial curetting. Bimanual examination shows the uterus to measure 4 to 6 weeks, anteverted, smooth, mobile. Adnexa negative. Rectal declined. BUS within normal limits.

IMPRESSION: Clear cell carcinoma of unknown origin.

PLAN: Refer the patient to the University of Minnesota for diagnostic workup and treatment. The patient and University of Minnesota will be advised of the results of the biopsies when they become available.

PATHOLOGY REPORT LATER INDICATED: See Report 54.

21. OPERATIVE REPORT

PREOPERATIVE DIAGNOSIS: Atelectasis of the right lower lobe, suspecting either a mucous plug or obstructing cancer.

POSTOPERATIVE DIAGNOSIS: Mildly inflamed airways with some thick secretions. No definite mucous plug was seen, and certainly no cancer was noted.

PROCEDURE PERFORMED: Bronchoalveolar lavage, bronchial brushings, and bronchial washings.

For a detail of drugs used and amounts of drugs used, please refer to the bronchoscopy report sheet.

The patient was in the ICU on the ventilator, intubated, and so we simply used ICU sedation. We put the bronchoscope down the endotracheal tube. We could see the trachea, which appeared okay. The carina appeared normal. In the right and left lungs, all segments were patent and entered, and in the right lower lobe and middle lower lobe, there were increased, thick, tenacious secretions. No definite mucous plug. It did take a little suctioning to dislodge all of the mucus; however, it was not as bad as I thought it would be looking at the x-ray. The area was brushed, washed, and then, to be more specific, because of evidence on chest x-ray of something going on in the periphery, a bronchoalveolar lavage of the right lower lobe is performed. The patient tolerated the procedure well. Specimens were performed. Specimens were sent for appropriate cytological, pathological, and bacteriological studies, and we hope to be able to follow up on that tomorrow.

PATHOLOGY REPORT LATER INDICATED: See Report 66.

22. OPERATIVE REPORT

PREOPERATIVE DIAGNOSIS: Chronic adenotonsillitis.

POSTOPERATIVE DIAGNOSIS: Chronic adenotonsillitis.

PROCEDURE PERFORMED: Tonsillectomy and adenoidectomy.

OPERATIVE NOTE: The patient is a 15-year-old woman who was seen in the office and diagnosed with the above condition. Decision was made in consultation with the patient to undergo the procedure.

She was admitted through the same-day department and taken to the operating room, where she was administered general anesthetic by intravenous injection. She was then intubated endotracheally. The Jennings gag was inserted into the mouth and expanded; this was secured to a Mayo stand. Two red rubber catheters were placed through the nose and brought out through the mouth; these were secured with snaps. This was done to elevate the palate. A laryngeal mirror was placed in the nasopharynx. The adenoid tissue was visualized. Using suction cautery, the adenoid tissue was removed in systemic fashion. Once this was completed, the red rubbers were released and brought out through the nose. The right tonsil was grasped with an Allis forceps and retracted medially using a harmonic scalpel, and the capsule was entered bilaterally. The tonsil was removed from its fossa in an inferior, and one small area was cauterized. The left tonsil was then grasped with an Allis forceps and retracted medially. Again, the capsule was identified laterally, and the harmonic scalpel was used to remove the tonsils from its fossa in an inferior to superior fashion. Once this was completed, the bed was inspected, and two small areas were cauterized here. Three tonsillar sponges were soaked in 1% Marcaine with epinephrine; one was placed in the nasopharynx, and one in each tonsil bed. These were left in position for 5 minutes, and at the end of this interval they were removed. The beds were inspected. No further bleeding was noted. The gag was then removed from the mouth. The TMJ joint was checked. The patient was allowed to recover from a general anesthetic and taken to the post anesthesia care unit in stable condition. There were no complications during this procedure.

PATHOLOGY REPORT LATER INDICATED: Benign tonsil and adenoid tissue.

23. OPERATIVE REPORT

PREOPERATIVE DIAGNOSIS: Pleural fluid, unknown cause.

POSTOPERATIVE DIAGNOSIS: Loculated pleural effusion with removal of 40 cc of bloody pleural fluid.

PROCEDURE PERFORMED: Diagnostic thoracentesis.

On ultrasound, the areas were loculated by that method as well as by attempting to draw out fluid. I had to do four different sticks to get 40 cc of fluid and that was about the extent of each pocket. There were four different pockets I entered just in the one general area that was marked by ultrasound. This, of course, was done after marking it with ultrasound, rubbing the area with swabs to sterilize the area, and then using 20 cc of 1% lidocaine for local anesthesia. With a one-pass maneuver, we were able to get into some fluid. At first actually, we did not get any fluid. We moved over about 1 inch, and then we were able to get 10 cc of fluid before the pocket petered out. The next one we got 5 cc, and I had to go to a different pocket to get that. Then in the fourth pocket we were able to get two syringe fulls with 10 cc to get at least 40 cc of fluid. As this was such a tenuous area, I did not put a chest tube in to drain it because I did not think we would get anything that would amount to anything with the small chest tube I had at my command. I think we might need thoracoscopy to break up adhesions and drain it right. Of course, the differential of bloody pleural fluid includes tuberculosis, trauma, cancer, and pulmonary embolus. A V/Q scan would probably be pointless in this particular effort. I think I would wait to see what the cultures are before I went down the pulmonary embolus tree. I will have to get a hold of Dr. Marrot about CT surgery.

PATHOLOGY REPORT LATER INDICATED: See Report 67.

24. OPERATIVE REPORT

PROCEDURE PERFORMED: Fiberoptic bronchoscopy, bronchial biopsy, bronchial washings, bronchial brushings.

PREPROCEDURE DIAGNOSIS: Abnormal chest x-ray

POSTPROCEDURE DIAGNOSIS: Inflammation in all lobes, pneumonia. With pleural plaquing consistent with possible candidiasis.

The patient was already on a ventilator, so the ET tube was introduced through the endotracheal tube. We saw 2.5 cm above the carina of the trachea, which was red and swollen, as was the carina. The right lung—all entrances were patent, but there were all swollen and red, with increased secretions. The left lung was even more involved, with more swelling and more edema and had bloody secretions, especially at the left base. This area from the carina all the way down to the smaller airways on the left side had shown white plaquing consistent with possible candidiasis. These areas were brushed, washed, biopsied. A biopsy specimen was also sent for tissue culture, as well as two biopsy specimens sent for pathology. Sheath brushings were also performed. The patient tolerated the procedure well, was still in the ICU, monitored throughout the procedure.

25. CARDIAC CATHETERIZATION REPORT

PROCEDURES PERFORMED: Left-sided heart catheterization, selective coronary angiography, and left ventriculography.

INDICATION: Chest pain and abnormal Cardiolite stress test.

COMPLICATIONS: None.

RESULTS:

I. HEMODYNAMICS: The left ventricular pressure before the LV-gram was 117/1 with an LVEDP of 4. After the LV-gram, it was 111/4 with an LVEDP of 10. The aortic pressure on pullback was 111/17.

II. LEFT VENTRICULOGRAPHY: The left ventriculography showed that the left ventricle was of normal size. There were no significant segmental wall motion abnormalities. The overall left ventricular systolic function was normal with an ejection fraction of better than 60%.

III. SELECTIVE CORONARY ANGIOGRAPHY:

A. RIGHT CORONARY ARTERY: The right coronary artery is a medium to large size dominant artery that has about 80 to 90% proximal/mid eccentric stenosis. The rest of the artery has only mild surface irregularities. The PDA and the posterolateral branches are small in size and have only mild surface irregularities.

B. LEFT MAIN CORONARY ARTERY: The left main has mild distal narrowing.

C. LEFT CIRCUMFLEX ARTERY: The left circumflex artery was a medium size, nondominant artery. It gave rise to a very high first obtuse marginal/intermedius, which was a bifurcating medium size artery that has only mild surface irregularities. The second obtuse marginal was also a medium size artery that has about 20 to 25% proximal narrowing. After that second obtuse marginal, the circumflex artery was a small size artery that has about 20 to 30% narrowing, a small aneurysmal segment. After that, it continued as a small third obtuse marginal that has mild atherosclerotic disease.

D. LEFT ANTERIOR DESCENDING CORONARY ARTERY: The left anterior descending artery was a medium size artery that is mildly calcified. It gave rise to a very tiny first diagonal that has mild diffuse atherosclerotic disease. Right at the origin of the second diagonal, the LAD has about 30% narrowing. The rest of the artery was free of significant obstructive disease. The second diagonal was also a small caliber artery that has no significant obstructive disease.

CONCLUSION:

1. Normal overall left ventricular systolic function
2. Severe single vessel atherosclerotic heart disease

RECOMMENDATIONS: Angioplasty stent of the right coronary artery.

26. CORONARY ARTERY BYPASS SURGERY

PREOPERATIVE DIAGNOSIS: Atherosclerotic heart disease coronary artery disease with depressed LV function.

POSTOPERATIVE DIAGNOSIS: Same.

PROCEDURE PERFORMED: Single vessel coronary artery bypass grafting, LIMA to LAD, off-pump.

ANESTHESIA: General endotracheal.

SPONGE COUNT, NEEDLE COUNT, INSTRUMENT COUNT: Correct.

ESTIMATED BLOOD LOSS: Approximately 666 cc and CellSaver given back is approximately 287 cc.

DRAINS: Four 19-French round Blake drains, one in the left chest, one in the right chest, one over the heart and one over the pericardial well, placed to Pleur-evac suction.

INDICATIONS: The patient is a 62-year-old man who has undergone approximately 12 heart catheterizations in the last several years. He has had recurrent in-stent stenosis of the proximal LAD lesion and also a branch of an OM with disease proximally. The patient is taken to the operating room because of recurrent angina, Class III anginal symptoms.

PROCEDURE: After informed consent was obtained, the patient was taken to the operating room. The patient was properly identified. A right and Swan-Ganz catheter was placed. A right arterial line was placed. A Foley catheter was inserted. The patient was prepped from his chin to both feet bilaterally. A midline sternotomy was performed. The sternum was divided with the sternal saw and the left internal mammary was harvested in a standard fashion.

Simultaneously, the right greater saphenous vein was harvested beginning in the thigh and extending down to the level of the knee. The vein was adequate for bypass grafting. It was excised. The wound was then closed in layers.

Once the LIMA was nearly completely dissected free, the patient was heparinized. The LIMA was divided distally and noted to have excellent flow. It was tied distally. LIMA bed was examined for bleeding. There appeared to be no bleeding present from the LIMA bed. Attention was then turned to the pericardium. The pericardium was opened. Pericardial stay sutures were placed. The left side of the pericardium was fashioned so that the LIMA could sit nicely to the LAD under the lung. Deep pericardial stitch was placed allowing the heart to be elevated and brought medially. A stay suture was placed around the proximal LAD and around the distal LAD. The octopus stabilizing device was used to stabilize the LAD at its mid portion. The proximal stay suture was placed down on the LAD. The LAD was opened and the LIMA had been fashioned for the anastomosis and the LIMA to LAD anastomosis was carried out using a 7-0 Prolene in a continuous running fashion using a single knot technique. LIMA pedicle was then sutured down. There appeared to be no leak present from the LIMA anastomosis. The starfish stabilizing device was placed on the apex of the heart. The heart was elevated. The lateral wall of the heart was examined extensively for the OM branch that had some proximal disease in it. This artery was not able to be identified. The heart was covered heavily in fat making it somewhat more difficult but a thorough examination was carried out. At this point I actually broke scrub, went to the catheterization laboratory, re-examined the heart catheterization and then went back to the OR again looking for that vessel. It almost could have been acting like a high diagonal vessel as it was a high OM but again in this territory in this distribution I could not identify that vessel, so only a single vessel LIMA to LAD anastomosis was created and the patient ended up with a single bypass. I think he should do well with just a single bypass.

The surgical sites were all examined for bleeding and there appeared to be no bleeding present. The patient was reversed with 50 mg of Protamine and four Blake drains were placed, one in the left chest, one in the right chest, one over the heart and one in the pericardial well. The patient tolerated the procedure well. The preoperative and postoperative transesophageal echocardiogram looked fine. Sternal wires were placed and then the wound was closed in layers. Initial cardiac index here revealed a cardiac index of approximately 2.4 on low dose nitro drip.

27. OPERATIVE REPORT

PREOPERATIVE DIAGNOSIS: Symptomatic right internal carotid artery stenosis.

POSTOPERATIVE DIAGNOSIS: Symptomatic right internal carotid artery stenosis.

OPERATIVE PROCEDURE:

1. Right carotid thromboendarterectomy with patch placement.
2. Intraoperative electroencephalogram monitoring.

INDICATION: This 30-year-old woman has a tight right internal carotid artery stenosis. She has had an episode of amaurosis fugax. She has some other medical problems that also complicate her overall situation, but she has a significantly tight stenosis that is symptomatic, and I would recommend an endarterectomy for this. The procedure, along with the risks, has been previously discussed with the patient. Please see the clinic notes. We will be doing this with the patient awake. We also will be doing EEG monitoring though because of the patient's overall condition, and if she does not end up needing to be intubated during the middle of the case, we will still be able to monitor her brain activity.

PROCEDURE: This was done with the patient under cervical block. Local anesthesia was also infiltrated (0.5% Marcaine with epinephrine). Dissection was carried down through a cervical oblique incision along the anterior border of the sternocleidomastoid muscle. Dissection was carried down to the carotid artery. The common carotid as well as the internal and external carotid arteries and superior thyroid arteries were all dissected free sharply and circumferentially controlled with vessel loops. The common carotid was controlled with umbilical tape and Rumel tourniquet. The patient was systemically heparinized. ACTs were obtained and followed. The ICA was occluded, then the common and then the external carotid. Arteriotomy was made. The plaque was hemorrhagic and ulcerated. It was quite friable. We were able to dissect this out with Freer elevator. This came out quite nicely. The distal endpoint feathered off nicely, but we did place one single tacking suture at the 6 o'clock position. This was 7-0 Prolene. We then used the Impra carotid patch to close the arteriotomy site. This was done with a CV-7 Gore-Tex suture in a running fashion. We heparinized, backbled, and forebled. Intermittently, we had her move her left hand during the case. After suturing the suture line, we opened up the external carotid and the common carotid. After about 10 heartbeats, we then opened up the internal carotid artery. There was bleeding from needle holes. This was controlled with FloSeal. There was good flow through all the arteries at the end of the procedure by Doppler. A 10-mm flat Jackson-Pratt drain was placed before closure of the wound. Hemostasis was present. At the end of the procedure in the admit room, she was awake and following commands and moving all of her extremities. She went to the recovery room in stable condition. I met with the patient's family postoperatively to discuss the operation.

ADDENDUM: It should be noted that this procedure was done with intraoperative EEG monitoring. No changes were noted in the EEG during the procedure. Clamp time was 40 minutes. A patch closure was used as noted. She was also reversed with 40 mg of prednisone at the end of the procedure.

28. OPERATIVE REPORT

INDICATION: Prolonged fetal heart rate deceleration.

PROCEDURE: Vacuum assisted vaginal delivery.

COMPLICATIONS: Shoulder dystocia, relieved with McRobert's maneuver.

PREAMBLE: The patient is a 33-year-old gravida 3, para 2, 38 week, 3 days gestation, admitted for induction secondary to pelvic pain. The patient received Pitocin and had artificial rupture of membranes and with this was able to progress to complete dilation. She then began pushing and some prolonged fetal heart rate decelerations down to about 90 beats per minute were noted. Because of this, a decision was made to proceed with vacuum extraction to assist in expediting delivery.

PROCEDURE NOTE: Maternal bladder was emptied using straight catheter. Pelvic examination was carried out and the cervix was confirmed to be fully dilated. Fetal vertex was present at +1 station. The small kiwi cup vacuum was then applied to the fetal vertex. On the second pull, there was one pop off but this was after good descent of the fetal head had been achieved. Baby then delivered and was a live-born male infant. There was some moderate shoulder dystocia present and this was relieved with McRobert's maneuver. The baby was handed off to the NICU team and is currently in the NICU for further observation. Apgar's are not available at this time. Cord blood gas is also pending.

There was a small second degree perineal tear. This was repaired using 3-0 chromic in usual manner. The patient tolerated this procedure well. Estimated blood loss during delivery was 200 cc.

29. OPERATIVE REPORT

PREOPERATIVE DIAGNOSIS:

1. Intrauterine pregnancy, 39 weeks.
2. Multiparity.
3. Desires permanent sterilization.
4. History of previous cesarean section times two.

POSTOPERATIVE DIAGNOSIS:

1. Intrauterine pregnancy, 39 weeks.
2. Multiparity.
3. Desires permanent sterilization.
4. History of previous cesarean section times two.

PROCEDURE: Repeat low transverse cervical segment cesarean section with postpartum tubal ligation.

ANESTHESIA: Spinal

ESTIMATED BLOOD LOSS: 800 cc

URINE OUTPUT: 40 cc

FLUIDS: 3000 cc

COMPLICATIONS: None.

FINDINGS: Viable male infant weighing 6 pounds 10 ounces with Apgars of 9 at 1 minute and 10 at 5 minutes.

PROCEDURE: The patient was prepped and draped in a supine position with left lateral displacement of the uterine fundus. Under spinal anesthesia and Foley catheter indwelling, a transverse incision was made in the lower abdomen using the old scar. The fascia was divided laterally. Rectus muscles were divided in the midline. The peritoneum was entered in a sharp manner. The incision was extended vertically. The bladder flap was created using sharp and blunt dissection and reflected inferiorly. The uterus was entered in a sharp manner in the lower uterine segment, and the incision was extended laterally with blunt traction. The head was delivered, the infant was delivered, and the bulb suctioned while the cord was being doubly clamped and divided. The infant was given to the intensive care nursery staff in good condition. The placenta was manually expressed. Uterus was delivered through the abdominal cavity and placed on a wet lap sponge. A dry lap sponge was used to ensure that the remaining products of conception were removed. The cervical os was ensured patent with a ring forceps. The uterus incision was closed with 0 Vicryl in an interlocking suture in two layers with second layer imbricating the first. Figure-of-eight sutures were also placed as required for hemostasis. Operative site was inspected, irrigated, and hemostatic. The bladder flap was reapproximated using 2-0 Vicryl in a continuous suture in the midline. The left tube was identified in its entirety, including the fimbriated and was grasped at its midportion and elevated. The mesosalpinx was transected using the Bovie. Approximately 3 cm of tube was isolated and excised. The proximal end of the distal portion and the distal end of the proximal portion were ligated with 0 chromic suture. Operative site was inspected and was hemostatic. Uterus was placed back in the midabdominal cavity. Pelvic gutters were irrigated. The anterior peritoneum was reapproximated with 2-0 Vicryl continuous suture. The incision was irrigated. Subcutaneous drain was placed, and the skin was closed with 2-0 silk. Sponges and needles were accounted for at the completion of the procedure. The patient left the operating room in apparent good condition after tolerating the procedure well. The Foley catheter was patent and draining a small amount of clear urine at the completion of the procedure.

30. OPERATIVE REPORT

PREOPERATIVE DIAGNOSIS: Complicated pregnancy with prior cesarean sections.

POSTOPERATIVE DIAGNOSIS: Complicated pregnancy with prior cesarean sections.

PROCEDURE PERFORMED: Amniocentesis for fetal lung maturity.

INDICATIONS: The patient is at $38\frac{1}{2}$-weeks' gestation and has had three prior C-sections and hospitalizations for recurrent episodes of pyelonephritis. We desired to check fetal maturity so we could expedite delivery if possible.

PROCEDURE: The patient was scanned with ultrasound, and few pockets were noted; therefore, we elected to do a suprapubic tap. The abdomen was prepped and draped. Dr. Marco elevated the breech of the infant up out of the pelvis, and we scanned suprapubically and found a nice pocket. A single tap was done and 10 cc of clear yellow fluid obtained. This fluid was checked for pH and was deeply blue on Nitrazine, indicating it to be most likely amniotic fluid, not urine. She tolerated this well.

31. OPERATIVE REPORT

Colonoscopy and Polypectomy

PREOPERATIVE DIAGNOSIS: Hematochezia.

POSTOPERATIVE DIAGNOSIS: Two small polyps in the cecum ascending colon, hot biopsied off. A small rectal polyp, hot biopsied off.

INDICATION: This is a 46-year-old white male with Tourette's and some MR who has had some hematochezia. There are no risk factors with no other symptoms.

PREOPERATIVE MEDICATIONS: Fentanyl 100 mcg IV; Versed 4 mg IV.

FINDINGS: The Pentax video colonoscope was inserted without difficulty to the cecum. The ileocecal valve was identified. The appendiceal orifice was seen. I could not enter the cecum. Just above the valve, there was a small 2 to 3 cm polyp. This was hot biopsied off. There was a sessile 3-mm polyp in the proximal ascending colon, hot biopsied off. Inspection of the remainder of the ascending colon, hepatic flexure, transverse colon, splenic flexure, descending colon, and sigmoid colon, revealed no erythema, ulceration, exudate, friability, or other mucosal abnormalities. The rectum showed a small 2-mm polyp that was hot biopsied off. The patient tolerated the procedure well.

IMPRESSION: Three small polyps, two in the cecum ascending colon area and one on the rectum, hot biopsied off.

PLAN: If these polyps are adenomatous, the patient should return again in 5 years for surveillance.

PATHOLOGY REPORT LATER INDICATED: See Report 56.

32. OPERATIVE REPORT

PREOPERATIVE DIAGNOSIS: Nonhealing duodenal ulcer.

POSTOPERATIVE DIAGNOSIS: Nonhealing duodenal ulcer.

PROCEDURES PERFORMED:

1. Exploratory laparotomy.
2. Partial gastrectomy (antrectomy).
3. Truncal vagotomy.
4. Gastrojejunostomy.
5. Cholecystectomy with intraoperative cholangiogram.

INDICATION: The patient is a 60-year-old female who presented with a nonhealing gastric ulcer. She has had symptoms for about a year. She complains of epigastric pain. Medical therapy with Prilosec failed, as did therapy for *H. pylori*. Biopsy of the ulcer has been done, and it was benign. The patient had a negative workup for gastrinoma. Calcium level was also normal. The patient now presents for exploratory laparotomy and partial gastrectomy. The risks and benefits were discussed with the patient in detail. She understood and agreed to proceed.

PROCEDURE: The patient was brought to the operating room. Her abdomen was prepped and draped in a sterile fashion. A midline umbilical incision was made. The peritoneal cavity was entered. Initial inspection of the peritoneal cavity showed normal liver, spleen, colon, and small bowel. There was an ulcer along the first portion of the duodenum just beyond the pylorus with some scarring. There was also an ulcer in the posterior part of the duodenal bulb, which was penetrating to the pancreas. We started dissection along the greater curvature of the stomach. Vessels were ligated with 2-0 silk ties. There was an enlarged lymph node along the greater curvature of the stomach, which was sent for frozen section. It proved to be a benign lymph node. This was the only enlarged node found during dissection. We then proceeded with truncal vagotomy. The anterior vagus and posterior vagus were identified. They were clipped proximally and distally, and a segment of each nerve was excised and sent for frozen section, and a segment of both vagus nerves was excised and confirmed by frozen section. An incision was made around the gastrohepatic ligament. The mesentery along the lesser curvature of the stomach was dissected. The vessels were ligated with 2-0 silk ties along the lesser curvature of the stomach. A Kocher maneuver was performed to aid mobilization. The pancreas was completely normal. No masses were found in the pancreas. There was penetration of the ulcer in the superior part of the head of the pancreas. Dissection was continued posterior to the stomach. The adhesions posterior to the stomach were taken down. The ulcer was in the posterior segment of the duodenal bulb just beyond the pylorus and it had penetrated the pancreas. All the posterior layer of the ulcer that was left adherent to the pancreas was shaved off. The stomach was divided with the GIA stapler so that the complete antrum would be in the specimen. The duodenum was divided between clamps. The stomach pylorus and first part of the duodenum were sent to pathology for examination. Then the duodenal stump was closed with running suture. Using 3-0 Lembert sutures, the posterior wall of the ulcer was incorporated for duodenal closure. The base of the duodenum was rolled over the ulcer, and it was all-incorporating to the duodenal closure. Our next step was to proceed with cholecystectomy. The gallbladder was separated from the liver, reflected, and taken down, and the gallbladder was divided from the liver with blunt dissection and cautery. The cystic artery was doubly ligated with silk. The cystic duct was identified. The cystic duct and gallbladder junction and gallbladder ducts were identified. Intraoperative cholangiogram was performed showing free flow of bile into the intrahepatic duct and into the duodenum. No leaks were seen. The cystic duct was doubly ligated, and the gallbladder was sent to pathology. The staple line in the proximal stomach was oversewn with 3-0 silk Lembert sutures. A retrocolic isoperistaltic Hofmeister-type gastrojejunostomy was performed on the remaining stomach and loop of jejunum. This was an isoperistaltic end-to-side two-layer anastomosis with 3-0 chromic and 3-0 silk. The stomach was secured to the transverse mesocolon with several interrupted silk sutures to prevent any herniation along the retrocolic space. The anastomosis had a good lumen and good blood supply. There was no twist along the anastomosis. Before the anastomosis was finished, a nasogastric tube was placed along the afferent limb of the jejunum to decompress the duodenum and prevent blow out of the duodenal stump. Extra holes were made in the NG tube to provide adequate drainage. The anastomosis was marked with two clips on each side, and a Jackson-Pratt drain was placed over the duodenal stump. The peritoneal cavity was irrigated until clear. Hemostasis was adequate. The fascia was then closed with interrupted 0 Ethibond sutures.

Skin edges were approximated with staples. Subcutaneous tissues were irrigated before closure. Estimated blood loss throughout the procedure was 200 ml. IV fluids: 3400 ml. Urine output: 840 ml.

FINDINGS:

1. Non-healing benign ulcer in the posterior duodenal bulb penetrating into the head of the pancreas.
2. Partial gastrectomy (antrectomy performed) and excision of the pylorus, first portion of the duodenum along with ulcer.
3. Hofmeister-type retrocolic isoperistaltic gastrojejunostomy.
4. Posterior wall of the ulcer that was penetrating into the pancreas incorporated into closure of the duodenal stump.
5. Truncal vagotomy performed with intraoperative frozen section confirming both vagus nerves.
6. Cholecystectomy performed with normal intraoperative cholangiogram.
7. Jackson-Pratt drain placed over the duodenal stump.

The items that are to be coded are listed below:

Partial gastrectomy (antrectomy) with gastrojejunostomy

Truncal vagotomy

Cholecystectomy with intraoperative cholangiogram

PATHOLOGY REPORT LATER INDICATED: Tissue showed no evidence of carcinoma. The radiologist reported the x-ray with 74300.

33. OPERATIVE REPORT

PREOPERATIVE DIAGNOSIS: Fournier's gangrene.

POSTOPERATIVE DIAGNOSIS: Same.

PROCEDURES PERFORMED:

1. Exploratory laparotomy with gastrotomy and removal of gastric foreign body.

Placement of 18 French Moss gastrojejunostomy feeding tube.

Diverting end-sigmoid colostomy (Hartmann's procedure).

SURGEON:

ANESTHESIA: General.

INDICATIONS: This is a 33-year-old patient with Fournier's gangrene who presents today for a diverting colostomy due to wound cares and placement of a gastrostomy tube for help with further follow-up feeding. He presents today for exploration. The family understands the risks of bleeding, infection, and postoperative fluid collections and wishes to proceed.

PROCEDURE: The patient was brought to the operating room, placed under general anesthesia, and prepped and draped with Betadine solution. A midline incision was made with a #10 blade and dissection was carried down through subcutaneous tissues using electrocautery. The midline fascia was identified and divided. The posterior sheath and peritoneum were sharply incised, thus allowing entry into the peritoneal cavity. There was some free fluid within the peritoneal cavity but no evidence of any abnormalities. We first identified the stomach and could feel what we felt were some polyps in the stomach. We first placed concentric purse-string sutures along the greater curvature of the stomach, opened up the stomach, and then passed an 18 French Moss gastrojejunostomy tube but were unable to get it down through the pylorus. We could feel these multiple masses in the stomach. We tied the purse-string sutures and inflated the balloon. We then made a small opening in the stomach with electrocautery and retrieved about 20 large what appeared to be vegetable matter and partially digested peppers and pickles. We irrigated with saline and then were able to pass the Moss gastrojejunostomy tube, the distal end, down through the pylorus. We closed the gastrotomy with a running 3-0 Vicryl and an outer layer of 3-0 silk Lembert sutures. We irrigated this area well. We then identified the sigmoid colon, fired a TLC-75 stapler across the sigmoid/descending colon and then placed a 3-0 Prolene on the rectal stump. We divided the mesentery between right angle clamps and tied the pedicles with 3-0 silk ties. We had a previously marked stomal opening in the left lower quadrant. We grasped this with a Kocher clamp, made an elliptical incision around this, and then divided the anterior sheath of the rectus in cruciate fashion, divided through the rectus muscles, and then opened the posterior sheath and peritoneum. We brought the colon then through this area. There was good mobility of the colon, and the colon was viable. We then irrigated the abdomen with saline, and, once all sponge and needle counts were correct, we closed the midline fascia with a combination of interrupted 0 Vicryl and running 0 PDS. The skin was closed with skin clips. The staple line was then removed from the colon and the colostomy was matured with 3-0 Vicryl sutures. An appliance was placed. All sponge and needle counts were correct. He tolerated this well.

Prior to leaving the operating room, we took down the dressings of his right leg. There was good granulation tissue which was pink and viable, and we then re-dressed the wound and sent him back to the surgical critical care unit in critical but stable condition.

PATHOLOGY REPORT LATER INDICATED: Idiopathic gangrene.

34. OPERATIVE REPORT

PREOPERATIVE DIAGNOSIS: Severe internal and external hemorrhoids.

POSTOPERATIVE DIAGNOSIS: Same.

PROCEDURE PERFORMED: Three quadrant hemorrhoidectomy.

ANESTHESIA: Spinal.

INDICATION: This is a very pleasant female who presents with severe internal and external hemorrhoids who presents today for elective excision. She understands the risks of bleeding, infection, and postoperative fluid collection. She wishes to proceed.

PROCEDURE: The patient was brought to the operating room and placed under spinal anesthesia, prepped and draped sterilely with Betadine solution. Digital rectal examination was first performed. There were severe external hemorrhoids. Pratt anoscope was inserted. The severest of the hemorrhoids were at the 6 o'clock, 9 o'clock, and 3 o'clock positions. These were each grasped with an Allis clamp, excised in diamond shape fashion. The mucosal defects were closed with running locked 3-0 Vicryl with the suture lines imbricated with 3-0 chromic sutures. This gave us a good closure that was hemostatic. We anesthetized the area with 30 cc of 0.5% Sensorcaine with epinephrine solution and then placed four gauze in the rectal canal. She tolerated this well and was taken to recovery in stable condition.

PATHOLOGY REPORT LATER INDICATED: Benign tissue.

35. OPERATIVE REPORT

PROCEDURE: Placement of CORFLO, feeding tube.

INDICATION: Feeding, patient with gastroparesis.

PROCEDURE: The patient was placed in the sitting position and then tilted to the right with a wedge. CORFLO was placed at the level of 19 cm without any complications. KUB was then done demonstrating the tip of the CORFLO in the third portion of the duodenum. After confirmation of postpyloric position of the CORFLO, the patient was started on Ultracal at 10 cc/hr.

36. OPERATIVE REPORT

PREOPERATIVE DIAGNOSES:

1. Expressed desire of the operating gynecologist to insert indwelling ureteral stents for ease of dissection of the anticipated enlarged adherent uterus.
2. Gynecologic diagnosis of pelvic endometriosis.

POSTOPERATIVE DIAGNOSES: Same.

PROCEDURE PERFORMED: Cystourethroscopy, insertion of bilateral ureteral catheters.

PROCEDURE: After general anesthesia and after the abdomen and genitalia had been prepped and draped in the usual fashion, the patient was placed in the dorsolithotomy position. The genitalia were examined and proved to be essentially unremarkable. The urethra was instrumented with a no. 24 French panendoscope sheath, and, using the foroblique and right-angle lenses, inspection of the entire vesical cavity showed no indication of any pathologic lesion. There is slight indention and some of the bladder incident to the uterine impression. The two ureteral orifices appear to be essentially unremarkable. The left ureteral orifice was catheterized with a no. 6 French Whistle Tip catheter with ease. The catheter was advanced to approximately 25 cm on the left side. Attention was then directed to the right side, and the right ureteral orifice was catheterized with a no. 6 French Whistle Tip catheter. The catheter was placed at approximately 24 cm. The bladder was then entered, Panendoscope sheath was withdrawn. A no. 18 French 5-ml balloon Foley catheter was then inserted into the bladder and left indwelling to the Foley catheter. The two ureteral catheters were anchored with no. 1 black silk. The two ureteral catheters and the Foley catheters were then connected to straight drainage and the patient was removed from the dorsolithotomy position. Dr. Weasly, the patient's gynecologist, then proceeded with a total abdominal hysterectomy and bilateral salpingo-oophorectomy.

37. OPERATIVE REPORT

PREOPERATIVE DIAGNOSIS: Recurrent transitional cell carcinoma of the bladder.

POSTOPERATIVE DIAGNOSIS: Same.

PROCEDURE PERFORMED: Cystoscopy; multiple random bladder biopsies.

CLINICAL NOTE: This patient has recurrent transitional cell carcinoma of the bladder. He has had BCG bladder instillation to help prevent recurrence. His last instillation was 6 weeks ago. The patient is doing well. He denied any complaints.

PROCEDURE: The patient was given a general endotracheal anesthetic and prepped and draped in lithotomy position. A 24 French resectoscope was passed into the bladder under direct vision. The urethra was normal. Prostate was non-obstructed. Inspection of the bladder demonstrated areas of hyperemia that would be most consistent with BCG changes but might also represent recurrent TCC. These areas were biopsied using a cold-cup biopsy. A 24 French resectoscope loupe was then used to cauterize these areas. Ureteric orifices were identified. Clear urine could be seen effluxing bilaterally.

The patient tolerated the procedure well. A B&O suppository was placed rectally after the end of the procedure. An 18 French Foley catheter was placed to straight drainage. Bimanual examination showed no significant abnormality and the prostate felt normal.

The patient will be scheduled for recheck cystoscopy in three months time providing pathology shows no evidence of recurrent tumor.

ADDENDUM: Total resected and fulgurated area of the bladder was 7 square centimeters.

PATHOLOGY REPORT LATER INDICATED: See Report 55.

38. OPERATIVE REPORT

PREOPERATIVE DIAGNOSIS: Urinary incontinence.

POSTOPERATIVE DIAGNOSIS: Same.

PROCEDURE PERFORMED: Insertion of double cuff artificial urinary sphincter with 25 cc reservoir (multi-component).

CLINICAL NOTE: This patient has had radiation for prostate cancer. This recurred. He then had cryotherapy. His PSA is undetectable but he has significant urinary incontinence unresponsive to pharmacotherapy. External clamp devices have been unsatisfactory.

PROCEDURE NOTE: The patient was given a spinal anesthetic, prepped and draped in a supine position. A penoscrotal incision was made. A 16 French Foley was placed in the bladder to straight drainage. The urethra was dissected to the level of the bulb. The bulbocavernous muscle was very atrophic and was not dissected off the urethra. A double cuff placement was selected. The urethra was mobilized in two places with a small bridge of tissue between them. These cuffs were incised. Both were incised at 4.5 cm. A reservoir space was created by manual dissection in the left inguinal canal into the retropubic space. The reservoir was placed, cycled, and filled with 25 cc of sterile saline. Both cuffs were placed in the usual fashion. The pump was then placed in the mid-scrotal pouch. Connections were made using a Y connector and straight connectors in the usual fashion. The system was cycled; it worked well. Foley catheter was withdrawn to insure cycling appropriately. Subcutaneous tissues were closed with 3-0 chromic and skin with a 4-0 subcuticular Vicryl stitch. The pump was cycled again and then deactivated; the Foley catheter replaced. The patient tolerated the procedure well and was transferred to the recovery room in good condition. The wounds were thoroughly irrigated with bacitracin solution.

39. OPERATIVE REPORT

PREOPERATIVE DIAGNOSIS: Morbid obesity.

POSTOPERATIVE DIAGNOSIS: Same.

PROCEDURES:

1. Laparoscopic Roux-en-Y gastrointestinal bypass.
2. Liver biopsy.

ANESTHESIA: General.

INDICATION: The patient is a 36-year-old female who presents with morbid obesity. She has gone to the seminars, and we have discussed laparoscopic Roux-en-Y gastrointestinal bypass along with the risk of surgery including bleeding, infection, leakage from the anastomoses, conversion to open procedure, postoperative stenoses of the anastomoses, or bowel obstruction. She understands and wishes to proceed.

PROCEDURE: The patient was brought to the operating room and placed under general anesthesia. A Foley catheter and orogastric tubes were inserted. She was prepped and draped sterilely with Betadine solution. A supraumbilical incision was made with a #15 blade, and dissection was carried down through the subcutaneous tissues bluntly. The patient had an incisional hernia from an old trocar port site. We placed our operative trocar into the abdomen, insufflated the abdomen. There was no damage to the underlying viscera. Under direct vision, we then placed two, midclavicular line, 12 millimeter ports that were just lateral and above the umbilical port. There was a right upper quadrant 12 millimeter port in the anterior axillary line and a left upper quadrant 5 millimeter port in the anterior axillary line. These were all placed under direct vision with no damage to the bowel. The patient had some adhesions of her gastrohepatic ligament to the liver. We took these down using the harmonic scalpel. We then entered the retrogastric space and placed our taut catheter behind the stomach. We then flipped the omentum up over the top of itself. We elevated the transverse colon and opened the transverse colon where we could see the drain. We identified the ligament of Treitz and fired an Endo-GIA stapler across the bowel, down from the ligament of Treitz. We fired an additional load across the mesentery. We then counted out 100 centimeters of bowel and then performed a stapled side-to-side functional end-to-end anastomosis by opening the bowel on the proximal and distal sides with the harmonic scalpel, firing two loads of the Endo-GIA stapler and closing the anastomosis with an Endo-GIA fired staple line. This gave us a nice anastomosis. We closed the mesenteric defect here with an Ethibond suture and fixed with Laparoties. We then sutured the proximal end to the catheter and flipped the mesentery back down. We then brought the bowel and the catheter up in retrogastric fashion. Next we identified the angle of His. We opened the angle of His, and we fired five loads of the Endo-GIA stapler across the stomach. We had blown up the 20 cc balloon and had about a 20 cc pouch. Once we had completely transected the stomach, we went above and placed the Bioenteric catheter within the gastric pouch. We passed the snare through it. We made a separate stab incision in the upper abdomen and passed the wire through. We then fed the anvil end of the CEA-21 stapler down through the back of the pharynx down through the esophagus and brought out through our gastric pouch. We then enlarged the left midclavicular line, abdominal port, and placed the CEA-25 stapler through here. We opened the staple line on the bowel that we had brought up after we had removed the taut catheter and placed the CEA stapler into the bowel, brought the spike through, connected the two ends of the CEA, closed it, and fired it. This gave us a nice 21 millimeter circular anastomosis. We completed the anastomosis with the Endo-GIA stapler. We imbricated the staple line with two Ethibond sutures, placed a wad of fat over the last to adhere the fat near our staple line. We tested the anastomosis with air with the bowel clamped, and there was no evidence of a leak. We then placed Hemaseel over this anastomosis, and then once again mobilized the mesentery. We then closed the mesenteric defect where the small bowel had gone in retrogastric fashion with the Ethicon Endo-suture. We once again placed Hemaseel on our small anastomosis. We placed 10 flat Jackson-Pratt drains near our GJ anastomosis which came on out the left side, and our ii which came out on the right side anastomosis. We removed the trocar ports under direct vision. We then extended our umbilical incision and reduced the umbilical hernia. We closed the fascial defect with interrupted 0 Prolene sutures. We anesthetized the wounds at all areas with a total of 60 cc of 0.50 percent Sensorcaine with epinephrine solution. We secured the drains in place with 0 silk sutures and then closed the skin with 3-0 Prolene sutures. Steri-Strips and sterile Band-Aids were applied. All sponge and needle counts were correct. We left the taut catheter and a Penrose drain in the left midclavicular line incision.

All sponge and needle counts were correct. She tolerated this well and was taken to recovery in stable condition.

PATHOLOGY REPORT LATER INDICATED: See Report 63.

40. OPERATIVE REPORT

HISTORY: This patient, who is unknown to me, reports working in the shop at his home grinding metal approximately 5 hours ago. He was wearing safety glasses, but he has noticed a foreign body in his right eye. He reports slight irritation to the eye. Denies blurred vision.

PHYSICAL EXAMINATION: PERLA, fundi without edema. There was no foreign body on lid eversion. Slit lamp shows a foreign body approximately 2 to 3 o'clock on the edge of the cornea. This foreign body appears metallic. There is very small area of rust around the site. Iris is intact. There are no cells in the anterior chamber. Fluorescein dye reveals uptake only over foreign body.

PROCEDURE: Two drops of Alcaine were used in the right eye. Foreign body was removed with an eye spud without difficulty. Slight orange discoloration at the base of cornea, but no definite rust ring visible.

IMPRESSION: Residual corneal abrasion.

DISPOSITION: Foreign body removed from right eye.

41. OPERATIVE REPORT

PREOPERATIVE DIAGNOSIS: Cervical spondylosis, C5-6, C6-7, with cervical discs.

POSTOPERATIVE DIAGNOSIS: Same.

PROCEDURE PERFORMED: Anterior discectomy and osteophytectomy at C5-6 and C6-7, with allograft fusion and Zephyr plating.

This case was monitored with sensory evoked potentials throughout the case. There were no changes.

PROCEDURE: Under general anesthesia, the patient was placed in the cervical outrigger. The neck was prepped and draped in the usual manner. An incision was made parallel to the sternocleidomastoid, and then we got onto the omohyoid and incised this. Then with sharp dissection we got onto the prevertebral fascia, but the Farley-Thompson retractor in, and then I was able to localize the C5-6 and C6-7 interspaces. The plan here was to get rid of the ridges, the disc, and to fuse and plate. The discectomies were done at C5-6 and C6-7. The ridges were removed, the discs were removed, and then the cartilaginous surfaces were prepared for reception of the bony fusion. At C6-7, a #8 trial was utilized and at C5-6 a #7 trial was utilized with bone. I took off the ridges, I took off the osteophytes, I removed the discs. I got down to the dura on both sides and was satisfied now that I could put the trial in and place the bone graft in. This was done at both levels. This having been done, they were countersunk and I then utilized a Zephyr plate from C5 down to C7 and put a screw into C6 as well. This done, a Hemovac drain was placed into the wound. Of course, the plate was locked, and we then closed the wound in layers utilizing 2-0 chromic on the platysma with 2-0 plain in the subcutaneous tissue and 3-0 nylon interrupted mattress sutures on the skin. A dressing was applied. The patient was to wear a collar in the postop period.

PATHOLOGY REPORT LATER INDICATED: Benign bone and tissue.

42. OPERATIVE REPORT

PREOPERATIVE DIAGNOSES:

1. Ptosis, right upper lid.
2. Loss of superior visual field secondary to #1.
3. Superior hemianopia secondary to #l, right eye.

POSTOPERATIVE DIAGNOSES: Same.

PROCEDURE PERFORMED: Fasanella-Servat procedure, right upper lid.

ANESTHESIA: General endotracheal.

INDICATIONS: This 57-year-old white female has had progressively drooping lid on her right for many years which has now reduced her superior visual field in the right eye and has actually limited her vision. After the prior approval and the photos and documentation were obtained, it was noted that the patient did have a 3 to 4 mm ptosis of the right upper lid and we would approach this with a Fasanella-Servat procedure. The risk of infection, hemorrhage and reoperations were discussed.

PROCEDURE: After the patient was placed under suitable general endotracheal anesthesia; the superior tarsal border was then marked with a marking pen and a 15 Bard-Parker blade cut down through skin to the muscle area. The lid was then everted on a Desmarres retractor and two curved mosquitos were then placed with the point central and pointing superiorly when the lid was everted. A 6-0 gut rapid absorbing suture was then started through the skin incision at the superior tarsal border and then a purse string was then woven along the curve tips and then the 3 to 4 mm resection was then obtained and then the serpentine 6-0 gut suture was then approximated without cutting it and brought out through the skin and tied. It was allowed to retract into the knot. There was no bleeding and there was no cut suture. Maxitrol ointment, a Telfa pad and patch was applied and the patient was sent to the recovery room. There were no complications.

43. OPERATIVE REPORT

PREOPERATIVE DIAGNOSIS: Lumbar radiculopathy secondary to herniated L5-S1 disk.

POSTOPERATIVE DIAGNOSIS: Same.

PROCEDURE PERFORMED: Right L5-S1 hemilaminectomy with excision of herniated L5-S1 disk.

PROCEDURE: The patient was taken to the operating room and placed under general endotracheal anesthesia. He was rotated into the prone position on chest rolls with arms extended over the head. The lumbar region was shaved, prepped, and draped in the usual sterile manner. The proposed vertical midline incision was infiltrated with lidocaine, with epinephrine. The skin was incised and sharp dissection carried through the subcutaneous tissues. The fascia was incised and subperiosteal dissection undertaken at L5-S1. The hemilamina of L5 was then removed in piecemeal fashion. This allowed evaluation of both the L4-5 disk as well as the L5-S1 disk. At L5-S1, moderate-sized disk herniation was immediately evident. The surrounding capsule was incised, and a large fragment of ligamentous degenerative disk was removed. The interspace was then probed, and all degenerative disk material was removed. On completion, the thecal sac and nerve root were noted to be well decompressed at L4-5. The L4-5 level appeared normal. Epidural space was lined with Surgicel and fat graft, and the wound closed in interrupted layers, with 4-0 Vicryl subcuticular stitch for skin. Steri-Strips and sterile dressing were applied to the wound. The patient tolerated the procedure well and was transferred to the recovery room in good condition.

PATHOLOGY REPORT LATER INDICATED: See Report 57.

44. OPERATIVE REPORT

PREOPERATIVE DIAGNOSES:

1. Left orbitonasal mass.
2. Dry eye syndrome
3. Pseudophakia, both eyes.
4. Computerized tomography confirmed tumor left orbital, left nasal side.

POSTOPERATIVE DIAGNOSES: Same with the addition of low-grade lymphoma, left orbit.

PROCEDURE: Anterior orbitotomy, debulking and biopsy.

ANESTHESIA: General endotracheal anesthesia.

INDICATION: This 81-year-old white woman has had a progressively enlarging mass of the left superior nasal orbit, which had become quite hard and is attached to the bone. CT shows there has been no bony invasion, and the brain has not been invaded. More than likely, this is a lymphoma but we want to take the patient for an anterior orbitotomy for debulking and biopsy.

DESCRIPTION OF PROCEDURE: After the patient was prepped and draped in the usual sterile fashion for ophthalmic surgery, the superior sulcus fold was marked out on her medial left upper lid. This was then cut through skin and muscle with the 25 Bard-Parker blade down through the orbital fat pad. It was noted there was some saponified fat and a hard mass that was kind of an orangish-red color and was attached to this. Two specimens were removed and tagged and sent for frozen section, and into the cryo unit with liquid nitrogen down to –80 degrees and was then brought in to remove the rest of the mass. There were some fragments of mass still attached to the nasal wall of the orbit. The frozen section revealed lymphoma, low grade, probably stage I, and since this is radiosensitive and that all of the tumor could not be removed without exonerating the orbit, it was elected to close at this point and treat the rest conservatively. The wound was closed after the remaining tumor was infiltrated with Solu-Medrol 125 mg per ml for a total of 2 ml, after which the wound was closed with interrupted 6-0 black nylon suture and Maxitrol ointment. Telfa pad, patch and shield were applied. The patient was sent to the recovery room. There were no complications.

PATHOLOGY REPORT LATER INDICATED: Lymphoma.

45. RADIOLOGY REPORT

EXAMINATION OF: Chest.

CLINCIAL SYMPTOMS: Chest pain.

Portable Chest, AP Sitting (one view), 4:45 PM: Comparisons are made with the previous study of 08/23/XX. The cardiac silhouette is not grossly enlarged for this projection. The mediastinum is not widened. Lung fields are generally clear and expanded to the periphery. Cardiac monitors do superimpose the chest.

CONLCUSION: Generally stable appearance of the chest, unchanged compared with the previous study.

46. RADIOLOGY REPORT

EXAMINATION OF: Biophysical profile.

CLINICAL SYMPTOMS: High blood pressure, estimated menstrual age 28 weeks 5 days.

BIOPHYSICAL PROFILE: The placenta is located along the anterior wall. It is heterogeneous in echotexture, grade II. The AFI is 5.4 cm, which is low. Fetal motion noted by the technologist. Heart rate 147 beats per minute. Intrauterine hypoechoic area seen anteriorly within the uterus measures about 2 cm in size and a second similar sized hypoechoic area is located within the uterus. Both findings are presumed fibroids.

   They are nonspecific findings, however. Biophysical profile was scored a perfect 8 out of 8.

47. CT SCAN

EXAMINATION OF: CT of orbits.

CLINICAL SYMPTOMS: Left eye pain.

CT OF ORBITS: CT of orbits in axial and coronal planes without contrast. Patient was vomiting therefore contrast was not given.

1. Complete opacification of right aspect of sphenoid sinus.
2. Near complete opacification of right maxillary antrum.
3. Polypoid membrane thickening left maxillary antrum.

4. Scattered membrane thickening throughout a few ethmoidal air cells.
5. Remainder negative.

48. MRA REPORT

EXAMINATION OF: MRA-brain.

CLINICAL SYMPTOMS: Third nerve palsy.

MAGNETIC RESONANCE EXAMINATION OF THE ARTERIAL VASCULATURE OF THE POSTERIOR FOSSA AND CIRCLE OF WILLIS REGION was performed utilizing three-dimensional time-of-flight multislab technique. Raw data and selected maximum-intensity projection images were photographed. Additionally, I have personally manipulated the maximum-intensity projections on a computer console in order to view the vasculature from various angulations.

I don't appreciate evidence of aneurysm. In particular, I don't appreciate evidence of aneurysm in the region of the posterior communicating arteries. I have personally reviewed the raw data images.

Bilaterally, there is some signal loss at the origin of the A1 segment of each anterior cerebral artery. This gives the appearance of stenosis. Most probably, this is technical, rather than due to true stenosis, but stenosis is not ruled out.

Internal carotid arteries appear unremarkable. Vertebral arteries are unremarkable. The basilar artery is unremarkable.

Proximal segments of the middle and posterior cerebral arteries appear unremarkable. Posterior communicating arteries are not visualized and are most probably very small.

49. RADIOLOGY REPORT

EXAMINATION OF: X-Ray Abdomen; single view.

CLINICAL SYMPTOMS: Malnutrition.

FINDINGS: A single supine view of the abdomen is submitted for interpretation. The majority of the pelvis and a portion of the left side of the abdomen are excluded from this examination. Feeding tube is identified. The tip overlies the left upper quadrant. Air is present within both small and large bowel which does not appear distended as visualized on this examination. There is degenerative change and dextroscoliosis of the lumbar spine. Surgical clips overlie the right upper quadrant. Opacity is noted in the left lung base which may relate to atelectasis or infiltrate. Followup is suggested.

50. RADIOLOGY REPORT

EXAMINATION OF: Left foot.

CLINICAL SYMTPOMS: Severe foot pain.

TWO VIEWS, LEFT FOOT: Comparison is made with the most recent films available 10/15/XX. There is diffuse demineralization of the osseous structures of the foot. Soft-tissue swelling is seen. Erosive changes have been previously described involving multiple metatarsophalangeal joints, and these are identified once again today. The differential is not significantly changed compared with the previous examination.

IMPRESSION:

1. Overall there is no significant interval change compared with 10/15/XX. There are extensive demineralization and extensive erosive changes involving the metatarsophalangeal joints and digits as described previously. Large cystic lesion is identified within the calcaneus as previously seen.

2. Diffuse soft tissue swelling and inferior calcaneal spur.

51. CT REPORT

CT of Abdomen

CLINICAL HISTORY: Increased liver enzyme.

TECHNIQUE: The patient was scanned from the dome of the diaphragm through the iliac crest after administration of oral and intravenous contrast.

COMPARISON: Comparison is made with a previous ultrasound examination dated 11/18/XX.

FINDINGS: Evaluation of the liver demonstrates mildly decreased attenuation to be present throughout the liver diffusely. No focal abnormalities are present within the liver. The spleen, pancreas, kidneys, and adrenal glands appear unremarkable. No enlarged lymph nodes are seen within the abdomen. No abnormal fluid collections are seen within the abdomen. The lung bases appear clear. No pleural effusions are seen.

IMPRESSION:

1. There is diffusely decreased attenuation present within the liver. This suggests the presence of fatty infiltration of the liver. No focal abnormalities are seen within the liver.

2. The remainder of the CT examination of the abdomen appears unremarkable.

52. LUNG SCAN REPORT

EXAMINATION OF: Ventilation-perfusion lung scan.

CLINICAL SYMPTOMS: Shortness of breath.

VENTILATION-PERFUSION LUNG SCAN:

DOSE: 2.0 millicuries of technetium-99m DTPA via aerosol. 6.0 millicuries of technetium-99m MAA IV. Comparison is made with chest radiograph obtained at the same time.

There is inhomogeneity regarding ventilatory scan. This is seen bilaterally. There appears to be elevation of the right hemidiaphragm.

There is decreased perfusion and ventilation along the right posterior lung base. The patient is noted to have pulmonary opacities and pleural effusions on chest radiograph. Small area of decreased perfusion and ventilation noted along the posterior aspect of the left upper lobe. Overall findings indeterminate for pulmonary embolus.

IMPRESSION: Indeterminate probability for pulmonary embolus.

53. MRI REPORT

EXAMINATION OF: Myocardial perfusion imaging.

CLINICAL SYMPTOMS: Chest pain, shortness of breath.

Myocardial Perfusion Imaging: Cardiolite Heart Imaging: SPECT left ventricular myocardial perfusion imaging study was performed in this patient. 29.5 millicuries of technetium-99m sestamibi was injected intravenously at peak stress. The patient had a maximal heart rate of 88%.

Evaluation of the qualitative image series shows the left ventricular myocardium to have a normal uptake of tracer. There is no evidence to suggest myocardial infarction or stress-induced ischemia.

IMPRESSION: Normal Cardiolite heart imaging as described above.

54. FROM OPERATIVE REPORT 20

CLINICAL HISTORY: C/C clear cell CA pelvis.

SPECIMEN RECEIVED: A. Endocervical curettings. B. Endometrial biopsy.

GROSS DESCRIPTION:

A. The specimen is labeled with the patient's name and "ecc" and consists of specimen jar with negligible tissue. The specimen is filtered and placed in one cassette.

B. The specimen is labeled with the patient's name and "endometrial" and consists of approximately 1 cc of wispy fragments.

MICROSCOPIC DESCRIPTION:

A. Sections show no tissue after processing.

Sections show scant fragments of benign tissue consisting predominantly of endocervical tissue and lower uterine segment. The endometrial glands are lined by 1 to 2 layers of columnar epithelium. Neoplasia/hyperplasia is not seen.

DIAGNOSIS:

A. Endocervical curettings: No tissue for processing.

Endometrial biopsy: Scant fragments of benign endocervical mucosa and lower uterine segment; neoplasia not identified.

SPECIMEN RECEIVED: Pelvic mass biopsy.

GROSS DESCRIPTION: Received in a container labeled with the patient's name are three cylindrical tan-brown tissue segments measuring 1.5 to 1.7 cm and 0.1 cm. The specimen is totally submitted.

MICROSCOPIC DESCRIPTION: The needle biopsy of the pelvic mass tissue shows a tumor with sheets and nests of moderately pleomorphic enlarged cells with abundant cleared cytoplasm. Irregularly outlined hyperchromatic nuclei are present centrally or in eccentric positions within the cells. A prominent vascular supporting network extends through the tumor cell sites.

DIAGNOSIS:

Pelvic biopsy, needle biopsy: Metastatic clear cell carcinoma.

COMMENT: The above described morphology strongly suggests a renal clear cell carcinoma.

55. FROM OPERATIVE REPORT 37

CLINICAL HISTORY: Bladder cancer.

SPECIMEN RECEIVED: Random bladder biopsy.

GROSS DESCRIPTION: The specimen is labeled with "biopsy" and consists of three, 3 specimen is processed in toto in patient's name and random bladder pink-tan tissue biopsies in 1 cassette.

MICROSCOPIC DESCRIPTION: Sections show fragments of bladder mucosa showing vascularization and congestion with mild lymphocytic, plasma cell infiltrates and lymphoid aggregates. The urothelium varies from normal to moderate to severe dysplasia to carcinoma in situ with full thickness cytologic atypia and occasional mitoses. One fragment shows grade 2 papillary transitional cell carcinoma. The underlying lamina propria shows reactive fibroblasts with scattered lymphocytic, plasma cell and eosinophilic infiltrates with admixed multinucleated giant cells. No definitive stromal invasion is identified.

DIAGNOSIS:
Random bladder biopsies: Moderate to severe urothelial dysplasia/transitional cell carcinoma in situ and noninvasive grade 2 (of 3) papillary transitional cell carcinoma.

56. FROM OPERATIVE REPORT 31

CLINICAL HISTORY: Adenoma.

SPECIMEN RECEIVED: Cecal ascending polyp.

GROSS DESCRIPTION: Received in a container labeled "cecal ascending polyp" are three fragments of tan tissue measuring 0.3 to 0.4 cm diameter. The specimen is totally submitted.

MICROSCOPIC DESCRIPTION: The cecum and ascending mucosal fragments show glands that vary in size and configuration and are lined by uniform epithelial cells. Hyperplasia of the glandular and surface epithelium are prominent with serrated architectures evident.

DIAGNOSIS:
Cecum and ascending colon biopsies, mucosal (three): Hyperplastic polyps, (three).

57. FROM OPERATIVE REPORT 43

CLINICAL HISTORY: Lumbar herniated disk.

TISSUE RECEIVED: Lumbar disk.

GROSS DESCRIPTIONS: Submitted in formalin, labeled with the patient's name and "lumbar disk" are several irregular fragments of pink-tan ragged tissue measuring approximately 2 × 1.5 × 0.5 cm in aggregate. Submitted in toto.

MICROSCOPIC DESCRIPTIONS: The slide shows several irregular fragments of fibrocartilaginous intervertebral disk material. There are no significant inflammatory infiltrates or evidence of neoplasm.

DIAGNOSIS:
Intervertebral disc, lumbar region, diskectomy: fragments of intervertebral disk.

58. PATHOLOGY REPORT

SPECIMEN RECEIVED: A. polyps, cecum/sigmoid—adenoma. B. Barrett's esophagus—rule out dysplasia.

GROSS DESCRIPTION: The specimens are received in two containers:

A. In the container labeled "colon biopsy and polyp" are four fragments of tan-pink tissue measuring 0.3 to 0.6 cm diameter. The specimen is totally submitted as "A".

B. In the container labeled "Barrett's esophagus biopsy" are six fragments of tan-gray tissue measuring 0.1 to 0.3 cm diameter. The specimen is totally submitted.

MICROSCOPIC DESCRIPTION:

A. The mucosal fragments of the cecum and sigmoid colon show polypoid architectures with adenomatous features within surface and glandular epithelial sites. The glands vary in size and configuration and are lined by enlarged, mildly pleomorphic cells with elongated hyperchromatic nuclei.

B. The esophageal biopsies demonstrate gastric cardia mucosa exhibiting intestinal metaplasia. The glands vary in size and configuration and have uniform elongated epithelial cells. Separation by a fibrous lamina propria is evident.

DIAGNOSIS:

A. Cecum and sigmoid colon biopsies, mucosal: Adenomatous polyp fragments.

B. Esophageal biopsy: Gastric cardia mucosa with intestinal metaplasia, consistent with Barrett's esophagus.

59. FROM OPERATIVE REPORT 14

SPECIMEN RECEIVED: Muscle biopsy, left deltoid.

INDICATION: Lipoma left posterior axillary fold.

GROSS DESCRIPTION: Received in a container labeled "muscle biopsy left deltoid" is a fragment of brown tissue measuring $0.7 \times 0.5 \times 0.5$ cm. The specimen is totally submitted.

MICROSCOPIC DESCRIPTION: The skeletal muscle of the left deltoid shows normal morphology.

DIAGNOSIS:
Muscle biopsy, left deltoid: No pathologic diagnosis.

60. FROM OPERATIVE REPORT 7

CLINICAL HISTORY: Mass of axillary fold.

SPECIMEN RECEIVED: Lipoma from axillary fold.

GROSS DESCRIPTION: The specimen is labeled with the patient's name and "lipoma from axillary fold, intramuscular" which consists of a loosely encapsulated yellow adipose tissue, $8 \times 7.8 \times 1.8$ cm. Sectioning reveals homogeneous yellow adipose tissue throughout. Representative sections in 4 cassettes.

MICROSCOPIC DIAGNOSIS: Mature adipose tissue consistent with lipoma, axillary fold.

61. PATHOLOGY REPORT

CLINICAL DIAGNOSIS AND HISTORY: Cyst.

TISSUE(S) SUBMITTED: Lesion, back.

GROSS DESCRIPTION: Specimen is received in fixative and consists of a 3.3 × 2.5 × 2.2-cm thin-walled cyst containing charcoal, gray-black, friable material.

MICROSCOPIC DESCRIPTION: One microscopic slide examined.

DIAGNOSIS: Follicular cyst, infundibular type, skin of back.

62. FROM OPERATIVE REPORT 12

CLINICAL HISTORY: Left ischial ulcer.

SPECIMEN RECEIVED: Ischial tissue (left).

GROSS DESCRIPTION: Received in a container labeled "left ischial tissue" is an irregularly shaped fragment of soft tissue with a small portion containing an ellipse of skin. The specimen measures 18 × 7.5 × 6 cm in greatest dimension. The skin ellipse measures 4.5 × 2.5 × 0.3 cm. A central opening measuring 2 cm in greatest dimension is present. The remainder of the tissue has a nodular solid tan gray to brown appearance. On sectioning diffuse fibrosis extends through the area. Representative portions are submitted.

MICROSCOPIC DESCRIPTION: The soft tissue of the left ischial region demonstrates extensive diffuse fibrosis with mild infiltrates of mononuclear inflammatory cells. A significant portion of the soft tissue is covered with granular fibrin containing sheets of neutrophils that rest upon a granulation tissue base. The adjacent epidermis shows pseudoepitheliomatous hyperplasia and normal maturation pattern.

DIAGNOSIS: Skin and soft tissue of left ischial region, excision: Granulation tissue, extensive, with diffuse fibrosis and mild chronic inflammation. Ulcer with mild to moderate acute inflammation.

63. FROM OPERATIVE REPORT 39

CLINICAL HISTORY: Morbid obesity.

SPECIMEN RECEIVED: Liver biopsy.

GROSS DESCRIPTION: The specimen is labeled with the patient's name and "liver biopsy" and consists of a 2 cm needle core of greenish tissue.

MICROSCOPIC DESCRIPTION: Sections show liver showing mild fatty change. The portal triads are unremarkable.

DIAGNOSIS: Liver biopsy showing mild fatty change.

64. FROM OPERATIVE REPORT 6

CLINICAL DIAGNOSIS AND HISTORY: Cyst.

TISSUE(S) SUBMITTED: Scalp cyst.

GROSS DESCRIPTION: Specimen is received in fixative and consists of an ovoid, rubbery, gray-white, 2 × 1.3 cm diameter cyst with gray-white laminated, friable contents.

MICROSCOPIC DESCRIPTION: One microscopic slide examined.

DIAGNOSIS: Follicular cyst, isthmus-catagen type (pilar cyst), clinically scalp.

65. FROM OPERATIVE REPORT 19

CLINICAL HISTORY: Left upper lobe abscess—probably secondary aspiration, culture and pseudomonas.

SPECIMEN RECEIVED: Lung, left upper lobe.

GROSS DESCRIPTION: Received in a container labeled "left upper lobe of lung" is a lung upper lobe measuring 17 × 11 × 3.4 cm as a collapsed specimen. The lobe weighs 283 grams. All surfaces have a dull gray yellow exudate that extends over the pleura. The pleura has a wrinkled collapsed appearance. On sectioning the majority of the lung parenchyma is replaced by a necrotic collapsed cyst with a ragged gray-yellow wall. This completely encompasses the vast majority of lung parenchyma with only small portions persisting in the base of the upper lobe. Bronchus and vascular structures are identified and appear unremarkable. Multiple representative sections of lung parenchyma are submitted.

MICROSCOPIC DESCRIPTION: The left upper lobe tissue sections show an extensive area of coagulation necrosis and marked destruction of the pulmonary parenchyma. Sheets of neutrophils are present within fibrin and coagulation necrosis debris. The adjacent lung tissue shows collections of macrophages and inflammatory cells within alveoli. Abundant fibrin debris accompanies the inflammation. Prominent squamous metaplasia is present within the bronchial tree that persists. Extensive interstitial fibrosis within the adjacent lung parenchyma is also present.

DIAGNOSIS: Lung, left upper lobe, resection: Abscess, large, with severe acute inflammation and extensive necrosis. Interstitial fibrosis with chronic inflammation, adjacent lung tissue.

66. FROM OPERATIVE REPORT 21

CLINICAL HISTORY: Atelectasis lung.

GROSS DESCRIPTION: 20 ml of mucoid fluid received in one container.

SPECIMEN RECEIVED: Bronchial washing.

SPECIMEN ADEQUACY: Specimen satisfactory for cytologic evaluation.

DIAGNOSIS: Atypical cells, cannot rule out malignancy.

COMMENTS: Rare groups of mildly atypical squamous cells present, significance and origin unknown. Cytology correlated with accompanying histology specimen. Please see pathology report.
   Report amended due to transcription error on original. Discussed with Dr. Green.

67. FROM OPERATIVE REPORT 23

CLINICAL HISTORY: Pleural effusion, unknown cause.

GROSS DESCRIPTIONS: Ten ml bloody fluid received in one syringe.

SPECIMEN RECEIVED: Pleural fluid.

SPECIMEN ADEQUACY: Specimen satisfactory for cytologic evaluation.

DIAGNOSIS: No cytologic evidence of malignancy.

COMMENTS: Specimen shows predominantly lymphocytes.

68. 2/1/0X FAMILY PRACTICE SERVICE, MARK ADAMS, MD

(REPORTS 68 TO 79 ARE FOR THE SAME PATIENT)

This 68-year-old female presents to the office today requesting a complete physical examination. She recently moved to our area and states that she would like to establish with a family practitioner. She has a history of coronary artery disease, status post coronary artery bypass ×3 in 1978. She has been doing well. Gravid 3, para 3, postmenopausal about 20 years. History is also significant for hypertension, controlled by diet. Otherwise no complaints.

PAST MEDICAL HISTORY: Remarkable for conditions stated above.

OPERATIONS:

1. Hysterectomy with bladder repair, 1973
2. Bilateral blepharoplasty
3. D&C × 4

ALLERGIES: None.

MEDICATIONS: Digoxin 0.25 mg, Lasix 40 mg p.o. q.d., estrogen.

TOBACCO: Does not smoke.

ALCOHOL: Occasional.

SOCIAL HISTORY: Homemaker, mother of three. Husband recently transferred to area from California.

FAMILY HISTORY: Mother deceased from heart disease. Father has had multiple strokes. Two brothers, one with polio. Three children, health good. One sister, died of breast cancer at age 35.

REVIEW OF SYMPTOMS: Denies nausea, vomiting, headaches, dysuria, incontinence, dyspnea. Occasional bouts of atrial fibrillation; always converts spontaneously.

HEENT: Wears glasses. Otherwise negative.

RESPIRATORY: Negative.

CARDIOVASCULAR: Negative except as discussed above.

GI/GU: Postmenopausal, on estrogen.

ENDOCRINE: No diabetes or thyroid problems.

MUSCULOSKELETAL: Some arthritis, both hands.

PSYCHIATRIC: Negative.

PHYSICAL EXAMINATION: Reveals a very pleasant elderly female in no distress.

VITALS: Blood pressure is 140/84 right arm sitting position, 150/90 left arm sitting position; pulse 90 and regular.

WEIGHT: 115 lb.

SKIN: No skin lesions are present.

NODES: No lymphadenopathy.

ENT: Negative.

CHEST: Clear to auscultation.

CARDIAC: Reveals a regular rhythm. I did not hear any murmurs or gallops.

BREAST EXAMINATION: Right side free from lumps or masses. Small lump noted in left breast on examination, which is painless, without discharge, without retraction.

ASSESSMENT AND PLAN:

1. History of coronary artery disease, status post coronary artery bypass. No complaints at present, no abnormal findings. Continue medications as previously prescribed.

2. Breast mass on examination. Suggest mammography. If positive, consultation will be requested from surgery.

3. Postmenopausal, continue on estrogen therapy.

69. 2/2/0X JACOB BOND, MD

Patient has bilateral diagnostic mammography that shows normal finding on the right, but dense, suspicious area on the left. Suggestion by radiologist is further clinical study.

70. 2/5/0X JACOB BOND, MD

Patient is seen today in the clinic at the request of Dr. Adams for evaluation of suspicious lump in the left breast. Patient states that she does not practice self-breast examination and therefore was unaware of the existing lump. She does state, however, on reflection, that the left breast at times was painful. No nipple discharge or puckering has been noted. Patient states that she has a sister who died of breast cancer in her mid-thirties. No other family history for cancer was noted.

EXAMINATION: Both breasts seem to be symmetrical. No abnormal findings on first view, right breast examination benign. Left breast identifies small lump where calcifications were noted on mammography.

ASSESSMENT: Left breast mass.

PLAN: Although it is difficult to say that this is not a single cyst, I would recommend a breast biopsy at patient's earliest convenience to rule out any possible malignancy. Options to include conservative measures of waiting for further signs, repeat mammography, 6-month breast checks were discussed with patient as well as risks and benefits of biopsy and possible mastectomy if findings are positive. Patient wishes to discuss with her husband and will let me know what she decides.

Thank you for allowing me to participate in the care of Mrs. Smith. My recommendations are as above. I will await her further decision if she wishes further care from a surgical standpoint.

71. 2/8/0X JACOB BOND, MD

Phone call from patient wishing to schedule left breast biopsy. Scheduled for 2/10/0X by Dr. Bond.

72. 2/10/0X JACOB BOND, MD

This patient is a 68-year-old female with chief complaint of left breast mass, admitted for left breast biopsy. The patient has a history of hypertension, coronary artery disease, and coronary artery bypass ×3. She also has a history of hysterectomy and is on estrogen therapy. She was in her usual state of health until a physical examination in early February, which revealed a small mass in the left breast. Mammography reportedly confirmed presence of mass and calcifications. Right breast exhibited no abnormal findings. The patient had menarche at age 12 and has given birth to three children. The patient has a family history positive for one sister with breast carcinoma. Medical history: as stated above for hypertension and CAD.

PHYSICAL EXAMINATION: Reveals a well-developed, well-nourished female in no apparent distress. The vital signs are stable, afebrile. The HEENT examination is within normal limits. The neck is supple, and the trachea is midline. No masses or adenopathy are present. The lungs are clear to auscultation and percussion. The cardiovascular examination is within normal limits. The left breast exhibits the presence of a small mass. The right breast is within normal limits. The right axilla is normal without adenopathy. The left axilla reveals small, less than 1 cm nonfixed, no matted lymph nodes. The abdominal examination is within normal limits. The rectal examination is normal, with guaiac-negative stool present in the vault.

ASSESSMENT: Left breast mass, admitted for breast biopsy and possible mastectomy.

73. 2/10/0X JACOB BOND, MD

Breast biopsy was performed; pathology report documented adenocarcinoma of left breast. Patient underwent surgery the same day for mastectomy.

74. 2/10/0X JACOB BOND, MD

PREOPERATIVE DIAGNOSIS: Carcinoma of the left breast.

POSTOPERATIVE DIAGNOSIS: Same.

PROCEDURE PERFORMED: Left total mastectomy and left axillary node dissection. (Note: This is a modified radical mastectomy.)

HISTORY: Patient underwent left breast biopsy for suspicious lesion 2/10/0X. Pathology report returned with diagnosis of adenocarcinoma of breast. Patient and her family discussed the benefits of the proposed total mastectomy and the risks, including death. Patient gives her understanding and agrees to proceed with the proposed procedure.

PROCEDURE: With the patient in the supine position under good general endotracheal anesthesia, a folded towel was placed beneath her left scapula and her left arm abducted on a pillow. She was prepped thoroughly with Betadine; the extent of her mastectomy incision was marked with a marking pen. We went about a half an inch superior and half an inch inferior to her most medial circummammary incision, and it was a transverse incision. The draping was completed with Minnesota Mining drape and sterile paper in the usual manner. The superior flap was raised first. Bleeders on the breast were clamped and bovied; small bleeders on the flap were clamped and tied with 3-0 silk. The superior flap was raised to the clavicle inferior to the rectus sheath, medially to the sternal border, and laterally to the latissimus dorsi. The breast was outlined with a bovie, and then the breast was removed medially and laterally. We were somewhat concerned about involving the pectoralis muscle here, but it did not, and we could not see any invasion to the pectoralis fascia. Perforators were clamped and oversewn with 2-0 silk figure-of-eights. Small bleeders on the pectoralis major were bovied. The breast was allowed to fall laterally. The clavipectoral fascia was taken down. There was an area of scar tissue on the superior lateral portion of the pectoralis major attached to the breast, and we thought this was in the area of the previous biopsy. We had to dissect this off sharply, and it did not appear to be a cancer. Then she had a lot of inflammatory tissue in the axilla, which was rather difficult to define, but we exposed the axillary vein, hemoclipped the small venous tributaries, and dissected the axilla down to the 7th rib, and then took the breast off the serratus by bovie; the lateral chest bleeders were clamped and tied with 3-0 silk. The axilla was inspected, and the long thoracic and thoracodorsal nerve was intact. We left the superior branch of the intercostal brachial. It was dry. The mastectomy site was lavaged out with a liter of sterile water. Small bleeders were bovied. Several bleeders on the flaps were clamped and tied with 3-0 silk. The chest tubes were placed in the axilla and over the pectoralis major and exited laterally inferiorly, and the flaps were brought together without any tension with pulley sutures of 2-0 silk; then the wound was closed with a running 4-0 Prolene vertical mattress suture, removing the pulley sutures as we went. Vaseline dressings and dry dressings were applied.

Estimated blood loss was 400 ml. She tolerated this well. The flaps seemed to be intact. The drains were sewn into place and dry dressings applied. She tolerated the procedure well and was returned to the recovery room in good condition.

75. 2/12/0X JOYCE HARKNESS, MD, CONSULTING PHYSICIAN

CHIEF COMPLAINT: Atrial fibrillation.

Patient is a 68-year-old female, status post left total mastectomy for carcinoma of left breast. She has been doing fairly well postoperatively until this morning when she awoke with complaints of fluttering in the chest. ECG shows periods of rapid atrial fibrillation, with conversion to sinus rhythm spontaneously.

Past history is positive for CAD and hypertension. Patient is status post coronary artery bypass ×3. No chest pain or anginal symptoms have been noted.

Cardiac examination at present shows regular rate and rhythm; no gallops or murmurs are noted.

ASSESSMENT: Atrial fibrillation, status post left total mastectomy.

RECOMMENDATION: Treat conservatively with Coumadin at present. Monitor closely for signs of rhythm not converting spontaneously. Consideration would then have to be given to converting medically. Electrocardioversion is not recommended at this time.

76. 2/14/0X ANTHONY CASH, MD, CONSULTING PHYSICIAN

CHIEF COMPLAINT: Second-opinion surgery consultation (inpatient) regarding acute onset of no palpable pulses in lower extremities.

Mrs. Smith is a 68-year-old female with known history of CAD, status post coronary bypass in the 1970s. She recently underwent a total mastectomy 2/10/0X by Dr. Bond. Postoperatively, the patient has had an unremarkable course. Diet and activity were gradually increased. This morning she got up from bed about 4:30 and was weighed and had no problems. About 6:30 she suddenly experienced an acute onset of bilateral leg pain. The pain was excruciating. She was lying in bed when this first occurred. The surgical service was consulted about 7:30 this morning. By history from the patient, the pain gradually decreased. At the time of initial examination, she was complaining of a greater pain in her left thigh. She did state that her right leg had more of a numb feeling. She claimed that both legs were heavy feeling and that she would have to move every now and then to get relief from the pain.

Pertinent history reveals that the patient has been intermittently in atrial fibrillation. She has received two doses of Coumadin postoperatively for this atrial fibrillation.

Initial examination of the patient reveals a well-developed, well-nourished white female in no apparent distress. Heart: Regular rate and rhythm. Lungs are clear to auscultation bilaterally. Chest: The patient has a well-healing incision. There are no signs of infection, such as erythema or discharge. Abdomen: Positive bowel sounds, soft, nontender, nondistended. No rigidity on palpation. Examination of the pulses reveals the following: 2/4 in the radial, 2/4 in the carotid. No palpable pulses from the femoral on down. The patient does have dopplerable pulses in the femorals bilaterally. She has dopplerable left posterior tibial and no dopplerable right dorsalis pedis pulse. Neuro: Cranial nerves II–XII grossly intact.

IMPRESSION: Probable saddle embolus to the distal aorta.

PLAN: Patient in need of emergent embolectomy with possible aortofemoral reconstruction. Acute onset of bilateral leg pain and numbness. Embolism most likely from left atrium. Patient has been in and out of atrial fibrillation postoperatively. Discussed the risks, benefits, and complications of the procedure with the patient. The patient understands she will be cared for postoperatively in the surgical intensive care unit.

Thank you for this interesting consultation. We agree with your initial assessment and are happy to participate in the care of this nice lady.

77. 2/14/0X JACOB BOND, MD

PREOPERATIVE DIAGNOSIS: Saddle embolus, distal aorta.

POSTOPERATIVE DIAGNOSIS: Same.

PROCEDURE PERFORMED: Bilateral aortofemoral embolectomy via femoral artery approach, femoral embolectomy.

PROCEDURE: The patient was placed in the supine position and given a general anesthetic. She was prepped from her nipples to her toes. Following this, two bilateral groin incisions were made and dissection was carried down. The common femoral, profunda femoral, and superficial femoral arteries were identified on both sides and controlled with vessel loops. Following this, starting with the right side, a linear arteriotomy was made over the superficial femoral artery and profunda arteries. No. 3 Fogarty catheters were passed distally down the superficial femoral arteries and profunda arteries. No thrombus was recovered. They were then flushed with heparinized saline and controlled with vessel loops. Following this, no. 4 and no. 6 Fogarty catheters were sequentially placed up the common femoral artery toward the iliofemoral area. A lot of thrombus was removed, and good arterial inflow was established in the right leg. Before any arteriotomies had been made, the patient had been given 5000 units of IV heparin that had been given 5 minutes to circulate.

Following this, the arteriotomy on the right was closed with a running 5-0 Prolene suture. Before the arteriotomy was closed, it was back-flushed and fore-flushed. The clamps and vessel loops were all removed, and flow was restored to the right lower extremity. The patient had dopplerable posterior tibial pulses and palpable dorsalis pedis pulses at this point. Following this, a similar incision was made in the left lower extremity, and catheters were placed distally down the profunda and superficial femoral arteries, also flushing them sequentially with heparinized saline. No thrombus was removed from the distal arteries on the left; however, on the right, no. 4 and no. 6 Fogarty catheters were placed sequentially toward the iliofemoral artery and more thrombotic material was removed, restoring good arterial inflow. The arteriotomy on the left was closed in a similar fashion with running 5-0 Prolene. All the clamps were removed. There were palpable dorsalis pedis and dopplerable posterior tibial pulses at this junction of the procedure. Following this, both wounds were irrigated free of clot and debris. They were closed with three layers of interrupted 3-0 Vicryl, and the skin was closed with staples. The patient tolerated the procedure well and went to the recovery room in good condition.

78. 2/17/0X ERIC ARNOLD, MD, CONSULTING PHYSICIAN

REASON FOR CONSULTATION: Pleural effusion.

Patient is a 68-year-old female who was initially admitted for a left breast biopsy. Pathology confirmed carcinoma, and patient proceeded to have left total mastectomy. Hospital course has been complicated by atrial fibrillation and saddle embolism, requiring embolectomy. Patient is now 4 days postop embolectomy and has developed persistent pleural effusion. Attempts at medical management have failed, and patient is developing respiratory failure. A pleuracentesis is accomplished, with 500 ml of blood-tinged fluid immediately aspirated. Patient appears to receive immediate relief. Patient will be closely monitored in intensive care unit for additional signs of respiratory failure.

79. 3/10/0X JACOB BOND, MD

Patient in for follow-up appointment, as status post mastectomy on 2/10/0X. Hospital course was complicated by atrial fibrillation and embolism, requiring embolectomy. Patient also developed pleural effusion requiring pleuracentesis. Patient has now been discharged from the hospital for 10 days. Other than some incisional pain, patient seems to be doing well. No major complaints: denies shortness of breath, nausea, loss of appetite, fever, or pain in extremities. Energy levels seem to be returning to normal. Incision sites are examined, with no earythema or infection noted. Sutures are removed. Patient is instructed not to lift, push, or pull objects and to return to activities slowly. Wound care is reviewed. Patient is instructed to follow-up in 2 weeks or sooner if complaints.

80. PULMONARY FUNCTION STUDY

This 49-year-old presents with dyspnea. He has previous cigarette smoking history.

COMPLETE PULMONARY FUNCTION STUDY: Forced vital capacity is 4.87 L, 112% of predicted. FEV_1 is 4.02 L, 113% of predicted. FEV_1 is 83%. FEF 25% to 75% is normal. There is no significant response to bronchodilators. Flow volume loop shows a well-preserved inspiratory limb.

Total lung capacity by plethysmography is 6.82 L, 111% predicted. RV/TLC ratio and airway resistance are normal. Corrected DLCO was 18.99, 70% of predicted.

IMPRESSION:

1. Normal expiratory flow rates.
2. Normal lung volumes.
3. Mild reduction of DLCO is noted.

The cause of decreased diffusion capacity is unclear in this patient. Possible causes could include heart disease, pulmonary embolism, anemia, obstructive sleep apnea. Clinical correlation is advised for cause of abnormal diffusion. There is no evidence of coexisting obstructive or restrictive pulmonary disease.

Note: The items to be coded listed below:

- Spirometry before and after bronchodilator
- Respiratory flow volume loop
- Functional residual capacity
- Carbon monoxide diffusing capacity

81. OPERATIVE REPORT

PREOPERATIVE DIAGNOSIS: History of adenocarcinoma of the prostate.

POSTOPERATIVE DIAGNOSIS: History of adenocarcinoma of the prostate.

PROCEDURES PERFORMED:

1. Transrectal ultrasound performance with:
2. Volume study.
3. Needle localization.
4. Needle implantation
5. Cystoscopy.

ANESTHESIA: General.

ESTIMATED BLOOD LOSS: Minimal.

PROCEDURE: Please see the preoperative note for indications of the procedure, as well as full informed consent. The patient underwent a general anesthetic and was put in the extended dorsal lithotomy position. The table was decanted or in Trendelenburg 5 degrees. He was prepped and draped in the usual fashion, which included a 14-French Foley catheter with 120 mL of sterile saline in his bladder. The testicles and scrotum had been taped back and away. We irrigated the rectum with sterile saline, performing a pseudo-enema. The patient underwent transrectal ultrasound placement. This was connected to the gantry. The placement of ultrasound and the grid work were setup so that the base of the prostate is noted at #1 on the grid work. The anterior most component at approximately 4.5–5, prostate extended from side-to-side from a to F.

Five-mm increment imaging slices were obtained, starting at the base of the prostate, carrying it back for a total of 3 cm to 30. Volume of the prostate is approximately 33 mL.

The outline of the prostate was drawn during the volume study. This information was given to the computer electronically so that a plan could be developed. Once the plan had been completed, the placement of the needles was performed in the usual fashion. The dose was delivered via 125 seeds after placement of the needles.

The total number of needles was 41 for 107 seeds. The patient tolerated this well. At the conclusion, the patient was re-prepped and draped with the Foley catheter being removed and a cystoscopic evaluation was performed. There is no evidence of perforation of the urethra, bladder neck, or bladder. Urine within the bladder was clear. No seeds or spacers could be identified. An 18-French Foley catheter was then placed along with Triple antibiotic salve to the perineum and mesh panties. Her tolerated the procedure well overall. Estimated blood loss minimal.

82. OPERATIVE REPORT

PREOPERATIVE DIAGNOSIS: History of a nodular mass, mid-prostate with urinary retention.

POSTOPERATIVE DIAGNOSIS: History of a nodular mass, mid-prostate with urinary retention; possible macronodular prostate.

PROCEDURE: Cystoscopy, transurethral resection of the prostate.

ANESTHESIA: Spinal.

ESTIMATED BLOOD LOSS. Approximately 100 mL.

FINDINGS: Benign prostatic hypertrophy type changes.

This is an 76-year-old gentleman who has a history as outlined in the preoperative note. Cystoscopically there is a large, red, macronodular area along the base of the prostate, which has been noted. The patient is having outlet obstructing symptoms. He has some decompensation in his urinary bladder but in discussion with the findings he wishes to go through the transurethral resection of prostate as outlined and discussed.

The patient underwent a spinal anesthetic, was put in the dorsolithotomy position, prepped and draped in the usual fashion. Cystoscopic evaluation reveals the 1-cm nodule along the base of the prostate. This appears more macronodular but is not really prostatic or is very minimally prostatic. It could represent a deteriorating median lobe.

Resection of the prostate was started at the 12 o'clock position and was carried between 3 and 9 o'clock back to the plane of the verumontanum. The base tissue and the rest of the lateral walls were then resected. This was a pretty small prostate, around 20 ml of tissue. The area was separately resected.

At the conclusion of this procedure, the chips were irrigated out of the bladder. Final hemostasis was achieved. A #22 French 3-way Foley catheter was inserted, inflated, and irrigated with slightly tinged irrigant returning. He was taken to the Recovery Room in satisfactory condition.

83. OPERATIVE REPORT

PREOPERATIVE DIAGNOSIS: History of left cryptorchid testicle.

POSTOPERATIVE DIAGNOSIS: Left ectopic testicle.

PROCEDURE PERFORMED: Left groin exploration with orchiopexy.

ANESTHESIA: General.

Please see the preoperative note for indications of the procedure as well as full informed consent. This 14-year-old was recognized on a sports physical as having a non-palpable testicle. Through his younger years, it had been palpable.

The testicle on physical exam sat in the superficial inguinal canal next to the external ring. With him asleep, we went ahead and evaluated again and, again, the testicular cord was foreshortened, not allowing the testicle to get into the scrotum proper and sat slightly lateral ass noted on the preoperative note.

He underwent a general anesthetic as noted previously and was prepped and draped in the usual fashion. A transverse incision was made halfway between the anterosuperior iliac spine and pubic tubercle at the presumed location of the internal ring. The external oblique aponeurosis was opened along the course of its fibers to the external ring. The inguinal canal was opened. The external ilioinguinal nerve was identified and preserved. The testicle could be identified outside the inguinal canal lateral to it in its own small covering. This was opened and the cord, with the testicle, could be freed up. We removed some of the adhesions along the cord, which allowed very satisfactory length to allow it to fit well into the inferior aspect of the left hemiscrotum.

A separate incision was made in the left hemiscrotum. Subdartos pouch was formed using sharp and blunt dissection. The testicle was brought through in a medial tract performed by using blunt dissection with a hemostat. The testicle was brought down into the scrotum and out of the incision with ease. On the inferior pole of the testicle, a small 3-0 chromic was placed in the inferior most portion of the septum. The scrotal wall was then closed over the testicle with interrupted 3-0 chromic. Irrigation of the wound was performed. No active bleeding could be identified. The external oblique aponeurosis was closed utilizing 3-0 silk. Bupivacaine 0.25% without epinephrine was placed approximately 3 mL in the internal ring and 3 mL in the subcut. The subcut was closed with interrupted 3-0 chromic and 4-0 undyed Vicryl for subcuticular incision closure with Steri-Strips. He tolerated the procedure well.

84. TRANSURETHRAL NEEDLE ABLATION (TUNA) THERAPY

The procedure was performed in the usual fashion and multiple segments as noted.

Transrectal ultrasound was performed with the patient in the left lateral position. The ultrasound is performed in order to evaluate the prostate in detail, bladder neck, and seminal vesicles. Ultrasound shows a width of the prostate at 45 mm. The entire calculated volume of the prostate is approximately 40 cc's. Large amount of the bladder neck/median lobe is noted as prominent. No other findings are noted in the prostate.

A prostatic block was then performed. Using an 8", 18-gauge spinal needle, the area between the "angle" of the prostate to seminal vesicle laterally is identified. Needle is placed into position at that point under the rectum. 8 cc's of 2% Xylocaine are used to create the block.

The patient was then brought to the cystoscopic area. Further preparation includes viscous Xylocaine and liquid Xylocaine to the bladder. After a 15-minute wait, we proceeded with the procedure as follows.

The scope was advanced down into the urethra through the sphincter and prostatic urethra and into the bladder. A prominent bladder neck is noted. The length of the prostate is about 28 mm. The obstructing components are definitely the median lobe.

Treatments were performed utilizing a suggested needle-length of 16 mm. The treatments were performed 1 cm back from the bladder neck laterally. One cm back from that positioning, the next treatment halfway between the original and the verumontanum. This was performed bilaterally. All target temperatures were reached without difficulty. The fifth treatment zone was the median lobe. We retracted the needles to 12 mm to do this. The patient tolerated the procedure well. Foley catheter was placed at the conclusion of the procedure. Usual post procedure protocol to include antibiotics and pain relief medications.

85. OPERATIVE REPORT

PREOPERATIVE DIAGNOSIS: Glaucoma, open angle, right eye.

POSTOPERATIVE DIAGNOSIS: Same.

OPERATION PERFORMED: Sequential cyclocryotherapy, right eye.

INDICATION: This 74-year-old white female has an out-of-control glaucoma in her right eye. She is pseudophakic and has been allergic to multiple drops and has had one sequential therapy before that worked quite well and then she stopped taking her drops. It is obvious that despite the cyclocryotherapy, she will need to continue on the Pilocarpine.

DESCRIPTION OF PROCEDURE: After the patient was placed on the OR table, she was given a retrobulbar anesthesia of Xylocaine 2% with 0.75% Marcaine and Wydase for a volume of 3.5 cc. After this, she was prepped and draped in the usual sterile fashion for ophthalmic surgery and a wire lid speculum was used to separate the lids of the right eye. 3.5 mm from the limbus was marked out with a marking pen in the superior temporal quadrant and the right inferior nasal quadrant of her eye. The cryoprobe was liquid nitrogen and nitrous oxide and was applied to −80 for a 5-second treatment in a freeze-thaw-freeze triple row of cryotherapy laid down in both the defined quadrants. There were no complications. Maxitrol ointment, Telfa, and two pads were applied and the patient sent to the Recovery Room.

86. OPERATIVE REPORT

PREOPERATIVE DIAGNOSIS:
1) Blunt trauma with paint ball, right eye,
2) Hyphema, right eye, secondary to #1.
3) Recurrent hyphema, right eye, secondary to #1.
4) Corneal staining, right eye, secondary to #1.
5) Increased intraocular pressure, right eye, secondary to #l.
6) Dense cataract, right eye, secondary to #1.

POSTOPERATIVE DIAGNOSIS: Same.

PROCEDURE PERFORMED: Irrigation and aspiration of hyphema and blood clot anterior chamber, right eye.

ANESTHESIA: General endotracheal anesthesia.

INDICATION: This 14-year-old, white male has had persistent problems since he was hit with a paint ball in his right eye 2 weeks ago. It has not resolved. It has continued to bleed and now it has formed a huge clot. Because of the increase in pain and obvious corneal staining, it was elected to irrigate the clot at this time. No guarantees were made to the mother for vision.

DESCRIPTION OF PROCEDURE: After the patient was prepped and draped in the usual sterile fashion for ophthalmic surgery under general endotracheal anesthesia, a wire lid speculum was used to separate the lids of the right eye. The Super knife was then used in the limbal area to make a 2-mm–wide incision at the 8 o'clock meridian, and the chamber was filled with BSS Plus. Using the Simcoe I&A apparatus, gentle suction, and a push-pull method, the clot was removed and the blood was irrigated. There was no damage done to the lens surface or to the iris and the pupil remained round. Healon was used to help dissolve the clot and make it easier for aspiration. At the end of the procedure, all the Healon and blood clot was removed and the pupil remained round. There was a dense cataract well on its way to hyper-maturity already present, but no evidence of any vitreous or subluxation of the lens. The wound was closed with a 10-0 nylon suture, and the knot was buried. Healon was then placed over the cornea because the cornea showed some irregularity secondary to the paint ball explosion. Solu-Medrol was injected inferiorly Sub-Tenon's. Atropine 1% was placed in the eye and Maxitrol ointment and a Telfa pad, patch, and shield applied. The patient was sent to the Recovery Room. There were no complications.

87. OPERATIVE REPORT

PREOPERATIVE DIAGNOSES:

1. Cataract, right eye.
2. Pseudophakia, left eye.
3. Excess myopia, both eyes.
4. Diabetes mellitus.
5. Atrial fibrillation, controlled.
6. Hypothyroidism.
7. Pacemaker for history of bradycardia.

POSTOPERATIVE DIAGNOSIS: Same.

PROCEDURE PERFORMED: Extracapsular cataract extraction, right eye, with insertion of intraocular lens implant, right eye.

ANESTHESIA: MAC anesthesia.

INDICATION: This 86-year-old white female has had progressively decreasing vision in her right eye secondary to a nuclear sclerotic cataract that has reduced her vision to 20/400 which can be corrected to 20/100. She had successful cataract surgery in her left eye a year ago and has returned to 20/40 vision without glasses. She was counseled again as to the type of procedure, the need for medical clearance, anticoagulation regulation, and pacemaker regulation.

PROCEDURE: After the patient was placed on the OR table, she was given Nadbath and Van Lint anesthesia on a 25-gauge needle for a volume of 9 cc of Xylocaine 2% with 0.75% Marcaine and Wydase. The same mixture was administered on a blunt retrobulbar Atkinson needle for a volume of 4 cc without complications. After this, she was prepped and draped in the usual sterile fashion for ophthalmic surgery, and the Honan balloon was placed for four minutes by the clock at 35 mm Mercury. After this, the lid speculum was used to separate the lids of the right eye and a fornix-based flap was raised from 9 o'clock to 3 o'clock and the wet-field cautery was used. There was no excessive bleeding despite the use of the Coumadin. A 69 Beaver blade made a half-thickness O'Malley groove from 9:30 to 2:30 and the Super knife was used to enter the eye at 11 o'clock. The chamber was filled with Healon, and a dry, non-irrigating anterior capsulotomy was performed on a bent 25-gauge needle. The wound was extended with left and right corneal-cutting scissors, and three 8-0 Vicryls were post placed. Using a lens vectis, the nucleus was expressed without capsular rupture or iris prolapse. The post placed sutures were tied down and the Simcoe I&A apparatus was used to clean up excess cortex. It was noted that there was very weak zonular support and positive vitreous pressure. We elected at this point to fill the chamber with Healon, insert a lens glide, and a 14 diopter L122 UV lens was inserted. Miochol was used to bring down the pupil and eight 10-0 nylons were used to close the wound. A peripheral iridectomy was performed at 1 o'clock and there was no evidence of any vitreous. The Healon was left in the eye. The pupil was round and two 8-0 Vicryls closed the conjunctiva. Solu-Medrol was used sub-Tenon's inferiorly, and Pilopine gel, Maxitrol ointment, Telfa, two pads and an eye shield were applied.

There were no complications, and the heart rate was not out of ordinary since it was protected with a magnet.

88. OPERATIVE REPORT

PREOPERATIVE DIAGNOSES:

1. History of corneoscleral laceration, right eye.
2. History of retained sutures, right eye.

POSTOPERATIVE DIAGNOSIS: Same.

PROCEDURE PERFORMED: Removal of retained sutures, anterior cornea, right eye.

ANESTHESIA: General anesthesia.

INDICATIONS: This 17-year-old white male who suffered a severe injury to his eye with multiple lacerations of his right cornea has now recovered to the point that his vision is correctable with a contact lens to 20/25, however, there is a large amount of suture material, and it was elected to remove the sutures at this time.

PROCEDURE: After the patient was prepped and draped in the usual sterile fashion for ophthalmic surgery and he was under general anesthesia, the lid speculum was used to separate the lids of the right eye. Healon was placed over the sutures, a Super knife was used to cut them, and they were pulled with a combination of straight tiers and 0.12 forceps. One suture remained deeply buried and was left alone. None of the scleral sutures were removed. There were no complications and the chamber remained intact. He was patched with TobraDex ointment without Telfa for 24 hours, and we will make arrangements to see him within the week.

APPENDIX B

—

Answers to Workbook Questions

CHAPTER 1: INTRODUCTION TO THE CPT

Theory

1-4. any of the following: service or procedure, anatomic site, condition or disease, synonym, eponym, abbreviation

5. d
6. a
7. b
8. c
9. Radiology
11. American Medical Association, or AMA
13. stand-alone code
15. codes or CPT codes
17. 1966
19. Health Insurance Portability and Accountability Act, or HIPAA

Practical

21. **77799**
23. **77499**

Pathology and Laboratory

25. **81099**

Medicine

27. **96999**

CHAPTER 2: EVALUATION AND MANAGEMENT (E/M)

Theory

1. c
3. a
5. e
7. b
9. high
11. low
13. elements
15. moderate severity
17. self-limited/minor severity
19. contributory
21. medical record
23. subjective
25. consultation, attending
27. concurrent
29. review of systems

Practical

Office or Other Outpatient Services and Hospital Inpatient Services

31. a. minimal, minimal/none
    b. minimal
    c. straightforward
    d. **99201**
33. **99219** (Evaluation and Management, Hospital Services, Observation Care)
35. **99223** (Hospital Services, Inpatient Services, Initial Hospital Care)
37. **99231** (Hospital Services, Inpatient Services, Subsequent Hospital Care)

Consultation Services

39. **99243** (Consultation, Office and/or Other Outpatient) Note: All three key components must be met for the service to qualify for the higher level code. In this case, only the MDM complexity was of a higher level, requiring the choice of the lower level code.
41. **99253** (New Patient, Inpatient Consultations)
43. **99232** (Hospital Inpatient Services, Subsequent Hospital Care)
45. **99231** (Hospital Inpatient Services, Subsequent Hospital Care)
47. **99241** (Consultation, Office and/or Other Outpatient, New or Established Patient)
49. **99245** (Consultation, Office and/or Other Outpatient, New or Established Patient) Note: Normally this would be appended with a -32 modifier. However, it isn't listed since modifiers aren't covered until Chapter 3.

Emergency Department, Nursing Facilities, Domiciliary, and Home Services

51. **99282** (Emergency Department Services)
53. **99342** (Home Services, New Patient)

55. **99334** (Nursing Facility Services, Subsequent Care)
57. **99324** (Domiciliary Services, New Patient)

Prolonged Services and Case Management Services

59. **99205** for the office visit (Office and/or Other Outpatient Services, New Patient) and **99354** and **99355** for Prolonged Services (Prolonged Services)

Services from Throughout the E/M Section

61. **99205** (Office and/or Other Outpatient Services, Office Visit, New Patient)
63. **99234** (Discharge Services, Observation Care)
65. **99251** (Consultation, Inpatient)
67. **99291** (Critical Care Services, Evaluation and Management)
    99292 × 3 (Critical Care Services, Evaluation and Management)

Reports

69. Report 1: **99283** (Evaluation and Management, Emergency Department)
71. Report 3: **99212** (E/M, Office and Other Outpatient)
73. Report 5: **99232** (E/M, Hospital)

CHAPTER 3: ANESTHESIA SECTION AND MODIFIERS

Theory

1. moderate sedation
3. A
5. preoperative services
7. no

Practical

9. P4 (A patient with severe systemic disease that is a constant threat to life)
11. P3 (A patient with severe systemic disease)
13. P2 (A patient with mild systemic disease)
15. **01382 (Anesthesia, Knee)**
17. **00144 (Anesthesia, Corneal Transplant)**
19. **00124 (Anesthesia, Otoscopy)**
21. -50
23. -53
25. -32
27. -32
29. -76
31. -99
33. -55
35. -FA

Reports
37. Report 10: None, Only local anesthesia was used.
39. Report 15: **01820** (Anesthesia, Arm, Lower)
41. Report 28: **01960** (Anesthesia, Childbirth, Vaginal Delivery)

CHAPTER 4: INTRODUCTION TO THE SURGERY SECTION AND INTEGUMENTARY SYSTEM

Theory

General Medical Terminology
1. d
3. e
5. b

Matching Biopsy Specimens
7. c
9. a

Matching Procedures and Suffixes
11. l
13. c
15. d
17. h
19. a
21. j
23. o
25. i

Integumentary System Terminology
27. j
29. n
31. s
33. o or k
35. k or o
37. g
39. l
41. q
43. b

Practical

45. **12032** (Repair, Wound, Intermediate); **99070** Surgical tray (Special Services, Supply of Materials) Note: You do not code an E/M code because this is an established patient and the treatment constitutes the main service provided to the patient.

47. **19102** (Breast, Biopsy); **99070** Surgical tray (Special Services, Supply of Materials) Note: You do not code an E/M code because this is an established patient and the treatment constitutes the main service provided to the patient.

49. **11451** (Hidradenitis, Excision)
51. **11971** (Removal, Tissue Expanders, Skin)
53. **11975** (Insertion, Contraceptive Capsules)
55. **11444** for 4-cm of face and **11423-51** for 3-cm of neck (Skin, Excision, Lesion, Benign)
57. **17110** for the first lesion (Skin, Destruction, Benign Lesions)
59. **12035** for the 18.1-cm leg repair (Wound, Repair, Intermediate); **11040-51** (Debridement, Skin, Partial Thickness)
61. **17110** (Destruction, Warts, Flat)
63. **11100, 11101** × **2** (Debridement, Skin, Eczematous)
65. **16000** (Burns, Initial Treatment)
67. **19020** (Mastotomy)

Reports

69. Report 7: **21556** (Tumor, Thorax, Excision)
71. Report 9: **19120-RT** (Excision, Breast, Lesion)
73. Report 12: **15940** (Excision, Pressure Ulcer)

CHAPTER 5: MUSCULOSKELETAL SYSTEM

Theory

Musculoskeletal Terminology

1. d
3. j
5. b
7. c
9. h
11. g

Answer the Following

13. aspiration of a joint
15. fascia lata graft
17. arthroscopy
19. No, the removal is part of the cast service
21. The primary difference is extent. The codes in the musculoskeletal system subsection are of biopsies of muscle and/or bone, whereas the codes in the integumentary system subsection are for skin and subcutaneous tissue.

Practical

23. **29075** (Cast, Short Arm)
25. **28406** (Fracture, Calcaneus, with Manipulation)
27. **26700** (Metacarpophalangeal Joint, Dislocation, Closed Treatment)
29. **27520** (Fracture, Patella, Closed Treatment; without Manipulation)
31. **27570** (Manipulation, Knee)

33. **21343** (Sinuses, Frontal, Fracture, Open Treatment)
35. **20615** (Aspiration, Cyst, Bone)
37. **20822** (Replantation, Digit)
39. **20526** (Injection, Carpal Tunnel, Therapeutic)
41. **20665** (Removal, Fixation Device)
43. **21450** (Fracture, Mandible, Closed Treatment, without Manipulation)
45. **29750** (Cast, Wedging)
47. **29520** (Strapping, Hip)
49. **29220** (Strapping, Back)
51. **29049** (Cast, Shoulder)
53. **29860** (Arthroscopy, Diagnostic, Hip)
55. **29877** (Arthroscopy, Surgical, Knee)
57. **29848** (Ligament, Release, Transverse Carpal)
59. **21032** (Excision, Maxillary, Torus Palatinus)

Reports

61. Report 13: **20610-LT** (Injection, Joint Shoulder)
63. Report 15: **25606** (Fracture, Radius, Distal)
65. Report 17: **27244** or **27244-RT** (Fracture, Femur)

CHAPTER 6: RESPIRATORY SYSTEM

Theory

Respiratory Terminology
1. d
3. k
5. b
7. c
9. f
11. m
13. a
15. e

Answer the Following
17. nasal button
19. septoplasty
21. posterior
23. transtracheal and cricothyroid
25. -50

Practical

27. **31267** (Antrostomy, Sinus, Maxillary)
29. **31628** (Bronchoscopy, Biopsy), **31632** (Bronchoscopy, Biopsy) Note: Code 31628 is for a single lobe and two lobes were biopsied. Code 31632 is an add-on code reporting the biopsy of the other lobe.

31. **31575** (Laryngoscopy, Fiberoptic)
33. **30801** (Cauterization, Turbinate Mucosa) Note: Code specified unilateral or bilateral.
35. **30115** and **30115-50** (Excision, Nose, Polyp)
37. **31536** (Laryngoscopy, Direct)
39. **31400** (Arytenoidectomy)
41. **31720** (Aspiration, Trachea, Nasotracheal)
43. **31830** (Revision, Tracheostomy, Scar)
45. **32657** (Thoracoscopy, Surgical, with Wedge Resection of Lung)
47. **32800** (Hernia Repair, Lung)
49. **30930** (Fracture, Nasal Turbinate, Therapeutic)
51. **31613** (Tracheostoma, Revision)
53. **32440** (Pneumonectomy, Total)
55. **32900** (Resection, Ribs)
57. **32005** (Pleurodesis, Chemical)

Reports
59. Report 19: **32480** (Lobectomy, Lung)
61. Report 23: **32000** (Thoracentesis)

CHAPTER 7: CARDIOVASCULAR SYSTEM

Theory

Cardiovascular Terminology
1. n
3. g
5. m
7. c
9. v
11. o
13. p
15. e
17. l
19. k
21. y
23. b
25. r

Answer the Following
27. internally or externally, or intracardiac or external
29. epicardial and transvenous
31. no
33. -24
35. patient-activated event recorder
37. reversible
39. embolus

Practical

41. **33403** (Valvuloplasty, Aortic Valve)
43. **33464** (Valvuloplasty, Tricuspid Valve)
45. **93000** (Electrocardiography, Evaluation)
47. **92982** (Angioplasty, Coronary Artery, Percutaneous Transluminal)
49. **93010** (Electrocardiography, Evaluation)
51. **37609** (Ligation, Artery, Temporal)
53. **35452** (Angioplasty, Aorta, Intraoperative)
55. **33513** (Bypass Graft, Coronary Artery, Venous Graft)
57. **33967** (Balloon Assisted Device, Aorta)
59. **33641** (Heart, Repair, Atrial Septum)
61. **33533** (Bypass Graft, Coronary Artery, Arterial), **33517** (Coronary Artery, Bypass Graft, Arterial, Venous), **33530** (Reoperation, Coronary Artery Bypass, Valve Procedure)

Reports

63. Report 26: **33533** (Coronary Artery Bypass Graft (CABG), Arterial)

CHAPTER 8: FEMALE GENITAL SYSTEM AND MATERNITY CARE AND DELIVERY

Theory

Female Genital Terminology

1. d
3. h
5. b
7. m
9. c
11. j
13. f

Maternity Care and Delivery Terminology

15. e
17. g
19. f
21. j
23. l
25. o
27. i
29. n

Answer the Following

31. introitus
33. colpocentesis
35. false
37. colposcope
39. loop electrode excision procedure

41. hysterectomy
43. Radiology
45. Oviduct/Ovary
47. trimesters
49. estimated date of confinement
51. E/M

Practical

53. **57400** (Dilation, Vagina)
55. **56441** (Adhesions, Labial, Lysis)
57. **58558** (Hysteroscopy, Surgical with Biopsy)
59. **58920** (Ovary, Wedge Resection)
61. **58800** (Cyst, Ovarian, Incision and Drainage)
63. **59514** (Cesarean Delivery, Delivery Only)
65. **59020** (Fetal Contraction Stress Test)
67. **56440** (Marsupialization, Bartholin's Gland, Cyst)
69. **57065** (Destruction, Lesion, Vagina, Extensive)

Reports

71. Report 28: **59409** (Vaginal Delivery, Delivery Only) Note: You would bill the delivery only because by reading this note you have no idea if the delivery physician was her regular obstetrician for before and after delivery care.
73. Report 30: **59000** (Amniocentesis)

CHAPTER 9: GENERAL SURGERY I

Theory

Male Genital Terminology

1. c
3. e
5. b
7. d
9. e
11. f
13. i
15. c
17. c
19. a
21. f
23. a
25. d
27. e
29. a
31. d
33. c

Urinary System Terminology

35. j
37. a
39. b
41. e
43. i
45. h
47. g
49. k
51. j
53. c
55. l
57. e

Digestive Terminology

59. d
61. c
63. h
65. e
67. b
69. g
71. c
73. f
75. d

Mediastinum and Diaphragm Terminology

77. c
79. f
81. h
83. a
85. i
87. e

Practical

89. **50562** (Endoscopy, Kidney, via Incision)
91. **50760** (Ureteroureterostomy)
93. **42140** (Uvulectomy)
95. **43401** (Esophagus, Transection)
97. **44345** (Colostomy, Revision, Paracolostomy, Hernia)
99. **42104** (Excision, Ulvula)
101. **42831** (Adenoidectomy)
103. **49521** (Repair, Hernia, Inguinal)
105. **39520** (Hernia, Repair, Diaphragmatic)
107. **54650** (Orchiopexy, Abdominal Approach)
109. **40650** (Repair, Lip)
111. **42507** (Parotid Duct, Diversion)

113. **43605** (Biopsy, Stomach)
115. **44604** (Suture, Intestines, Large, Wound)
117. **49320** (Laparoscopy, Diagnostic)
119. **52283** (Urethral, Stricture, Injection, Steroids)
121. **54150** (Circumcision, Clamp or Other Device)
123. **54420** (Priapism, Repair, with Shunt)
125. **55860** (Prostate, Exploration, Exposure)
127. **54322** (Magpi Operation)
129. **54163** (Circumcision, Repair)
131. **50650** (Ureterectomy)

Reports

133. Report 31: **45384** (Colonoscopy, Removal, Polyp)
135. Report 33: **44143** (Colectomy, Partial, with Colostomy), **43500-51** (Gastrotomy)
137. Report 35: **43752** (Orogastric Tube Placement)
139. Report 37: **52240** (Cystourethroscopy, with Fulguration, Tumor)
141. Report 39: **43644** (Laparoscopy, Gastric Restrictive Procedures); **47001** (Biopsy, Liver)
143. Report 82 **52612** (Transurethral Procedure, Prostate, Resection)
145. Report 84 **53852** (Transurethral Procedure, Prostate, Thermotherapy, Radiofrequency)

CHAPTER 10: GENERAL SURGERY II

Theory

Hemic and Lymphatic Terminology

1. s
3. h
5. m
7. d
9. q
11. e
13. l
15. g
17. o
19. f

Endocrine System Terminology

21. c
23. f
25. d
27. g
29. h
31. b

Nervous System Terminology

33. g
35. h
37. b
39. d

Eye and Ocular Adnexa Terminology

41. c
43. d
45. e
47. g
49. o
51. p
53. u
55. n
57. l
59. r
61. t

Auditory System Terminology

63. g
65. n
67. h
69. i
71. k
73. a
75. c
77. l

Practical

79. **38720** (Lymphadenectomy, Radical, Cervical)
81. **38241** (Bone Marrow, T-Cell Transplantation)
83. **62256** (Removal, Shunt, Brain)
85. **68020**, **68020-50** or **68020-RT** and **68020-LT** (Incision and Drainage, Cyst, Conjunctiva)
87. **67938** (Removal, Foreign Bodies, Eyelid)
89. **69320** (Reconstruction, Auditory Canal, External)
91. **68520** (Excision, Lacrimal Sac)

Reports

93. Report 41: **63075** (Diskectomy), **63076** (Diskectomy), **22554** (Arthrodesis, Cervical Anterior, with Diskectomy), **22845** (Instrumentation, Spinal, Insertion), **20931** (Allograft, Spine Surgery, Structural), **95925** (Evoked Potential, Somatosensory Testing)
95. Report 43: **63030** (Hemilaminectomy)
97. Report 85 **66720** (Glaucoma, Cryotherapy)
99. Report 87 **66984** (Cataract, Removal, Extraction, Extracapsular)

CHAPTER 11: RADIOLOGY SECTION

Theory

1. c
3. b
5. a
7. b
9. f
11. a
13. e
15. i
17. h
19. j
21. c

Practical

23. **78499** (Nuclear Medicine, Heart, Unlisted Services and Procedure)
25. -26
27. **75705** (Angiography, Spinal Artery)
29. **70130** (X-Ray, Mastoids)
31. **70542** (Magnetic Resonance Imaging, Neck)
33. **73510** (X-Ray, Hip)
35. **75994** (Atherectomy X-Ray, Renal Artery)
37. **99219** for initial observation care (Evaluation and Management, Hospital Services, Observation Care); **70450** for CT Scan without mention of contrast (CAT Scan, without Contrast); **76516** for A-scan (Ultrasound, Eye, Biometry); **77261** for therapeutic radiation (Radiation Therapy Planning); **77402** for radiation delivery of single treatment area (Radiation Therapy, Treatment Delivery, Single); **77427** for weekly radiology therapy management (Radiation Therapy Treatment Delivery Weekly)
39. **76604** (Ultrasound, Chest); **71550** for the MRI (Magnetic Resonance Imaging, Chest); **33020** for the pericardiotomy (Pericardiotomy, Clot)
41. **73092** (X-Ray, Arm, Upper)
43. **77002** (Fluoroscopy, Needle Biopsy)
45. **76872** (Ultrasound, Rectal)
47. **72240** (Myelography, Spine, Cervical)
49. **70140** (X-Ray, Facial Bones)
51. **74010** (X-Ray, Abdomen)
53. **75870** (Venography, Sagittal Sinus)
55. **75945** (Ultrasound, Non-Coronary, Intravascular)

Reports

57. Report 45: **71010** (X-Ray, Chest)
59. Report 47: **70480-26** (CT Scan, without Contrast, Orbit)
61. Report 49: **74000-26** (X-Ray, Abdomen)

63. Report 51: **74160** (CT, with Contrast, Abdomen)
65. Report 53: **78464** (Myocardial, Perfusion Imaging)

CHAPTER 12: PATHOLOGY/LABORATORY SECTION

Theory

1. surgery
3. presence, amount
5. section
7. two, one for each specimen

Practical

9. **84520** (Urea Nitrogen, Quantitative); **84295** (Sodium); **84132** (Potassium); **82565** (Creatinine, Blood); **84550** (Uric Acid, Blood)*
11. **80076** (Blood Tests, Panels, Hepatic Function), **80061** (Blood Tests, Panels, Lipid Panel)
13. **80162** (Digoxin Assay)

Reports

15. Report 55: **88305** Urinary Bladder (Pathology, Surgical, Gross and Micro Exam)
17. Report 57: **88304** Intervertebral Disk (Pathology, Surgical, Gross and Micro Exam)
19. Report 59: **88305** Muscle (Pathology, Surgical, Gross and Micro Exam)
21. Report 61: **88304** Skin Cyst (Pathology, Surgical, Gross and Micro Exam)
23. Report 63: **88307** Liver (Pathology, Surgical, Gross and Micro Exam)
25. Report 65: **88309** Lung Lobe (Pathology, Surgical, Gross and Micro Exam)
27. Report 67: **88104** (Cytopathology, Fluids, Washings, Brushings)

CHAPTER 13: MEDICINE SECTION AND LEVEL II NATIONAL CODES

Theory

1. m
3. h
5. n
7. i
9. g
11. l
13. a
15. g
17. f
19. a

---

*Note: The Blood Urea Nitrogen (BUN) is part of the blood chemistry for this patient, and there is only one code for blood as the source of the sample—84520. Although there are other CPT codes to identify urea nitrogen, the source of the sample is the urine (84525-84545).

21. c

23. hearing test

25. stimulation of the cochlea to measure electrical activity

27. studying the capillaries of the eyes

29. a device for detecting color blindness

31. cornea and sclera together forming one organ

33. Temporary assignment codes used until a definitive decision can be made about appropriate code assignment (or similar wording)

35. no

37. drug codes

39. durable medical equipment

Practical

41. **95052 × 2** (Allergy Tests, Patch, Photo Patch)

43. **92341** (Spectacle Services, Fitting, Spectacles)

45. **92534** (Nystagmus Tests, Optokinetic)

47. **91034** (Esophagus, Acid Reflux Tests)

49. **90880** (Hypnotherapy)

51. **92626** (Rehabilitation, Auditory, Status Evaluation)

53. **90940** (Hemodialysis, Blood Flow Study)

55. **93503** (Catheterization, Cardiac, Flow Directed)

57. **94003** (Ventilation Assist)

59. **99144** (Sedation, Moderate)

61. **90471** (Administration, Immunization, One Vaccine/Toxoid), **90472** (Administration, Immunization, each additional Vaccine/Toxoid)

63. **11402** 1.2cm, back (trunk) (Excision, Skin, Lesion Benign); **A4550** (Surgical trays) or **99070** (Supply, Materials)

65. **99252** (Consultation, Inpatient), **E0180** (Pressure, Pad)

Reports

67. Report 68: **99204** (Office and/or Other Outpatient Services, New Patient) Note: no H/P examination, or MDC are specified.

69. Report 70: **99241** (Consultation, Office and/or Other Outpatient)

71. Report 72: **none**, as the admission is part of the surgical package

73. Report 74: **19307-LT** (Mastectomy, Modified Radical)

75. Report 76: **99253** (Consultation, Inpatient)

77. Report 78: **32000** (Thoracentesis)

79. Report 80: **94060** (Spirometry); **94375** (Pulmonology, Diagnostic, Flow-Volume Loop); **94240** (Pulmonology, Diagnostic, Functional Residual Capacity); **94720** (Pulmonology, Diagnostic, Carbon Monoxide Diffusion Capacity)

CHAPTER 14: AN OVERVIEW OF THE ICD-9-CM

Theory

1. a

3. f

5. a

7. h

9. j

11. d

13. b

15. f

17. c

19. a

21. g

23. d

25. true

27. true

29. reaction

31. obstruction

33. pregnancy

35. rapid

37. subcategory

39. category

41. subcategory

43. diagnosis code

45. procedure code

47. diagnosis code

CHAPTER 15: USING THE ICD-9-CM

Practical

1. **V18.1** (History [of], family, gout)

3. **V72.0** (Admission [for], vision examination)

5. **V73.4** (Screening (for), fever, yellow)

7. **V71.89** (Observation (for), suicide attempt, alleged)

9. **V04.1** (Vaccination, prophylactic, smallpox)

11. Nonunion of left tibia fracture (closed)

    Residual: nonunion fracture, **733.82** (Nonunion, fracture)

    Cause: fracture, tibia, **905.4** (Late effect[s] (of), fracture, extremity, lower)

13. Residual and cause: cerebrovascular accident, **438.21** (Late effect(s) (of), cerebrovascular disease with hemiplegia affecting dominant side)

15. **110.4** (Infection, fungus NEC, foot)

17. **601.0** (Prostatitis, acute); **041.00** (Infection, streptococcal NEC) in this order

19. **V55.3** (Colostomy, fitting or adjustment)

21. **V77.99** (Screening (for), immunity)

23. **272.2** (Hyperlipidemia, mixed)

25. **238.8** (Neoplasm, abdomen, uncertain behavior) ; **M8000/1** (Tumor, uncertain)

27. **211.5** (Adenoma, hepatocellular); **M8170/0** (Adenoma, hepatocellular, benign)

29. **250.71** (Diabetes, gangrene); **785.4** (Gangrene) in this order

31. **287.5** (Thrombocytopenia, thrombocytopenic)

33. **299.00** (Autism, autistic (child)(infantile))

35. **296.7** (Disorder, bipolar, atypical)

37. **038.0** (Septicemia, streptococcal (anaerobic))

39. **295.32** (Schizophrenia, paranoid)

41. **305.1** (Tobacco, abuse)

43. **300.01** (Disorder, panic)

45. **362.83** (Edema, retina)

47. **366.22** (Cataract, traumatic, total)

49. **389.10** (Loss, hearing, sensorineural)

51. **410.70** (Infarct, infarction, subendocardial)

53. **416.0** (Hypertension, pulmonary (artery), primary)

55. **427.0** (Tachycardia, paroxysmal, supraventricular)

57. **440.1** (Stenosis, renal artery)

59. **457.2** (Lymphangitis, chronic (any site))

61. **478.5** (Abscess, vocal cord)

63. **491.21** (Bronchitis, chronic, obstructive, with exacerbation (acute))

65. **528.2** (Stomatitis, aphthous)

67. **552.3** (Hernia, hiatal, with obstruction)

69. **571.6** (Cirrhosis, biliary)

71. **016.00** (Tuberculosis, abscess, kidney); **590.81** (Pyelitis, tuberculosis) Note: Code in this order.

73. **648.13** (Pregnancy, complicated by, hypothyroidism); **244.9** (Hypothyroidism (acquired)) Note: Code in this order.

75. **682.7** (Cellulitis, foot); **682.6** (Cellulitis, ankle); **041.10** (Infection, staphylococcal NEC)

77. **707.03** (Ulcer, decubitus, sacrum)

79. **705.83** (Hidradenitis)

81. **721.0** (Spondylosis; cervical, cervicodorsal)

83. **727.1** (Bunion)

85. **V30.01** (Newborn, single, born in hospital, with cesarean delivery or section); **749.20** (Cleft, palate, with cleft lip)

87. **789.1** (Hepatomegaly)

89. **791.0** (Proteinuria)

91. **783.5** (Polydipsia)

93. **810.00** (Fracture, clavicle)

95. **913.0** (Injury, superficial, elbow)

97. **850.9** (Concussion)

99. **924.01** (Contusion, hip)

101. **832.02** (Dislocation, elbow, posterior (closed))

103. **578.9** (Bleeding, gastrointestinal); **E935.6** (Table of drugs and chemicals, ibuprofen, therapeutic use)

105. a. Admission for dialysis and acute renal failure
    b. **V56.0** (Admission, for, dialysis, extracorporeal); **584.9** (Failure, renal, acute). It was not specified as "due to procedure," so you would not assign a complication from cardiac surgery code (997.5)

107. a. **965.09** (Table of drugs and chemicals, codeine, poisoning); **E850.2** (Table of drugs and chemicals, codeine, accident)
    b. **965.4** (Table of drugs and chemicals, acetaminophen, poisoning); **E850.4** (Table of drugs and chemicals, acetaminophen, accident)
    c. **980.0** (Table of drugs and chemicals, alcohol, grain, beverage, poisoning); **E860.0** (Table of drugs and chemicals, alcohol, grain, beverage, accident)
    d. **780.79** (Lethargy)
    e. **787.03** (Vomiting)
    f. **789.00** (Pain, abdominal)

109. **414.01** (Arteriosclerosis, coronary (artery), native artery); **496** (Disease, lung, obstructive (chronic)(COPD))

111. **482.41** (Pneumonia, due to, *Staphylococcus aureus*)

113. **045.02** (Poliomyelitis, cerebral), **784.49** (Dysphonia)

115. **922.32** (Contusion, buttock); **E885.9** (Slipping (accidental), on ice)

117. **197.6** (Ascites, malignant); **199.1** (Neoplasm, unknown site, primary)

119. **998.31** (Dehiscence, operation wound, internal)

121. **291.0** (Alcohol, delirium, tremors)

123. **370.24** (Keratitis, Welder's); **E926.2** (Radiation, light sources)

125. **382.9** (Otitis, media)

127. **360.63** (Foreign body, lens, retained or old)

129. **008.47** (Diarrhea due to Paracolon bacillus, NEC)

131. **V02.4** (Diphtheria, carrier (suspected) of)

133. **441.02** (Aneurysm, aorta, abdominal, dissecting)

135. **443.0** (Raynaud's, gangrene); **785.4** (Gangrene)

137. **451.11** (Thrombophlebitis, leg, deep (vessel), femoral vein)

139. **533.40** (Ulcer, peptic, with, hemorrhage)

141. **569.62** (Colostomy, malfunctioning)

143. **617.1** (Endometriosis, ovary); **617.3** (Endometriosis, round ligament)

145. **625.6** (Incontinence, urine, stress [female])

147. **786.50** (Pain, rib)

149. **684**, **373.5** (Impetigo, eyelid)
151. **756.52** (Marble, bones)
153. **715.33** (Osteoarthrosis, localized)
155. **518.5** (Distress, respiratory, adult syndrome (following shock, surgery, or trauma)); **E884.9** (Fall, from, off tree)
157. **381.62** (Obstruction, Eustachian tube (complete)(partial) cartilaginous, intrinsic)
159. **401.9** (Elevated, blood pressure)
161. **789.64** (Tenderness, abnormal)
163. **914.6** (Injury, superficial, hand); **E920.8** (Cut, cutting by, dart)
165. **944.20** (Burn, hands, second degree), 948.00 (Burn, extent (percent of body surface)
167. **943.20** (Burns, arm(s), second degree); **948.00** (Burn, extent (percent of body surface); **E924.2** (Burning, burns, hot, tap water)
169. **996.73** (Complications, due to, renal dialysis)
171. **915.6** (Injury, superficial, finger, not infected), **E920.8** (Cut, cutting by, splinter)
173. **275.0** (Hemochromatosis)
175. **V59.3** (Donor, bone, marrow)
177. **V55.3** (Attention to, colostomy); Note: Although not requested, the procedure code would be **46.52** (Closure, colostomy)
179. **790.22** (Findings, glucose, elevated, tolerance test)

Principal Diagnosis

181. Principal diagnosis and codes: Right orbital fracture, **802.6** (Fracture orbit, floor)

    Other diagnoses and codes:

    Right zygoma fracture **802.4** (Fracture, zygoma)

    Abrasion to head **910.0** (Injury, superficial, head)

    Assault by striking **E960.0** (Index to external causes, assault, brawl)

    Procedure: **76.79** Reduction Fracture, orbit, open (Index to procedures) and **76.92** implant (Implant, facial bone, synthetic)

Sequencing exercises

183. Principal diagnosis: cellulitis ankle or leg

    Other diagnoses: none
185. Principal diagnosis: colon cancer, primary malignancy

    Other diagnoses: bone cancer, secondary
187. Principal diagnosis: menorrhagia

    Other diagnoses: acute, bronchitis, canceled surgery

    Other diagnoses: second-degree burn thigh
189. Principal diagnosis: acute with chronic bronchitis

    Other diagnoses: none

Reports

191. Report 6: **709.2** (Scar); **86.3** (Excision, lesion, skin)
193. Report 8: **686.9** (Fistula, skin); **86.3** (Excision, lesion, skin)

195. Report 10: **952.00** (Injury, spinal cord, cervical C1-C4); **952.05** (Injury, spinal cord, cervical, C5-C7); **E819.9** (Accident, motor vehicle), **02.94** (Insertion, (skull, tongs)(with synchronous skeletal traction))

197. Report 12: **707.8** (Ulcer, face); **86.3** (Excision, lesion, skin)

199. Report 14: **781.99** (Symptoms, nervous system NEC); **83.21** (Biopsy, muscle)

201. Report 19: **513.0** (Abscess, lung); **32.3** (Lobectomy, lung, partial)

203. Report 28: **659.71** (Delivery, complicated (by), fetal heart rate or rythm); **660.41** (Delivery, complicated (by), dystocia, shoulder girdle); **664.11** (Delivery, complicated (by), laceration, perineum, second degree); **72.79** (Delivery, vacuum extraction); **73.09** (Rupture, membrane, artificial); **75.69** (Repair, perineum, laceration, obstetric (current))

205. Report 32: **532.70** (Ulcer, duodenum, chronic); Hospital: Procedure: **43.7** (Gastrectomy, with anastomosis, jejunum); **44.01** (Vagotomy truncal); **51.22** (Cholecystectomy); **87.53** (Cholangiogram, intraoperative)

207. Report 34: **455.3** (Hemorrhoids, external); **455.0** (Hemorrhoids, internal); **49.46** (Hemorrhoidectomy, by, excision)

209. Report 36: **617.3** (Endometriosis, peritoneal, pelvic); **59.8** (Insertion, ureteral stent); **57.32** (Cystourethroscopy)

211. Report 39: **278.01** (Obesity, morbid); **571.8** (Fatty, liver); **44.38** (Bypass, gastric, laparoscopic aspiration)(needle))

213. Report 42: **374.30** (Ptosis, eyelid); **368.40** (Defect, visual field); **368.46** (Hemianopia); **08.35** (Fasanella-Servat, operation)

215. Report 44: **202.81** (Lymphoma; lymph node of head, face, and neck); **375.15** (Syndrome, dry skin, eye); **V43.1** (Pseudophakia); **16.09** (Orbitotomy); **16.23** (Biopsy, orbit)

CHAPTER 16: THIRD-PARTY REIMBURSEMENT ISSUES

Theory

1. a. persons eligible for disability benefits from Social Security
   b. persons with permanent kidney failure

3. Social Security Administration

5. principal diagnosis, secondary diagnosis, procedures, age, sex, and discharge status

7. complication and comorbidity

9. 468, 476, and 477

11. 80%

13. 1 year

15. 90

17. 20%

19. October

21. Yale, late 1960s

23. sicker and more complex (either one or both)

25. Major diagnostic category

27. TEFRA

29. no